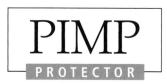

A Medical Reference Guide for Rotations

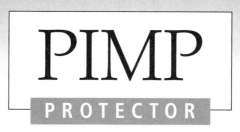

# PIMP
## PROTECTOR

**A Medical Reference Guide for Rotations**

## Quinn Holzheimer, D.O.

*Assistant Professor*
*Clinical Emergency Medicine*
*Georgetown University/Washington Hospital Center*
*Emergency Medicine Residency Program*
*Washington, D.C.*

Wolters Kluwer | Lippincott Williams & Wilkins
Health
Philadelphia · Baltimore · New York · London
Buenos Aires · Hong Kong · Sydney · Tokyo

*Acquisitions Editor:* Donna Balado
*Managing Editor:* Kelly Horvath
*Marketing Manager:* Jennifer Kuklinski
*Production Editor:* Gina Aiello
*Designer:* Steve Druding
*Compositor:* International Typesetting and Composition
*Printer:* R.R. Donnelly & Sons—Crawfordsville

Copyright © 2007
*Lippincott Williams & Wilkins; a Wolters Kluwer business.*

### DISCLAIMER

**Care has been taken to confirm the accuracy of the information present and to describe generally accepted practices. However, the authors, editors, and publisher are not responsible for errors or omissions or for any consequences from application of the information in this book and make no warranty, expressed or implied, with respect to the currency, completeness, or accuracy of the contents of the publication. Application of this information in a particular situation remains the professional responsibility of the practitioner; the clinical treatments described and recommended may not be considered absolute and universal recommendations.**

The authors, editors, and publishers have exerted every effort to ensure that drug selection and dosage set forth in this text are in accordance with current recommendations and practice at the time of publication. However, in view of ongoing research, changes in government regulations, and the constant flow of information relating to drug therapy and drug reactions, the reader is urged to check the package insert for each drug for any change in indications and dosage and for added warnings and precautions. This is particularly important when the recommended agent is a new or infrequently employed drug.

Some drugs and medical devices presented in this publication have Food and Drug Administration (FDA) clearance for limited use in restricted research settings. It is the responsibility of the health care provider to ascertain the FDA status of each drug or device planned for use in their clinical practice.

Library of Congress Cataloging-in-Publication Data

Holzheimer, Quinn.
    PIMP protector : a medical reference guide for rotations / Quinn
Holzheimer.
        p. ; cm.
    ISBN 0-7817-6999-X
    1. Internal medicine—Handbooks, manuals, etc.   2. Clinical clerkship
—Handbooks, manuals, etc.   I. Title.
    [DNLM: 1. Clinical Medicine.   2. Clinical Competence.
3. Students, Medical.    WB 102 H762p 2007]
    RC55.H595 2007
    616—dc22

                                                            2006029693

# Preface

"PIMPing," is the practice of resident or attending doctors presenting a set of very difficult questions to medical interns or students, who are expected to respond promptly and accurately. It's a time-honored tradition in the medical profession and has struck fear in the hearts of many a timid future doctor. *PIMP Protector* was written to guide you through this sometimes harrowing process. It's your best defense.

*PIMP Protector* features over (rounded 90) sections for the most common conditions you will see throughout your clerkships. Unlike other pocket reference guides that focus on only one topic, *PIMP Protector* will be useful on all of your clerkships. *PIMP Protector* also strips away the superfluous information that weigh down other less useful books. It is not necessary for you to know the dose of a heparin drip in pulmonary embolism, for example, but it is important for you to know the basic disease description, how to differential dyspnea, the pertinent positives and negatives in the history, the relevant physical exam findings, the appropriate lab tests to order, and its general treatment. This book also provides several concise "pearl" statements that are "universally PIMPed" as well as **current literature citations** that will allow you to quote a landmark journal article on the disease topic. Throughout the book are also helpful mnemonics, differential diagnosis tables, and frequently referenced information in easy-to-read chart format.

There will come a time on a new rotation where you will be asked to evaluate a patient who has a condition you are not familiar with. *PIMP Protector* will:

help you **confidently** and **comprehensively** evaluate and treat the patient;

give you the **foundation** to answer questions by your superiors;
**bolster** your knowledge in topics throughout your rotations; and guide you through your **day-to-day** referencing of high yield topics.

I wrote this book after years of being "PIMPed," and in my turn, "PIMPing" medical students, interns, and residents. There have been many times I was asked a question and did not know the answer, but did know where to find the information requested. I have also been in the situation where I did not ask for or look for certain information on the patient, leading to humiliating encounters with superiors. By reviewing the corresponding section in the *PIMP Protector*, you will have an excellent foundation for the disease process, will know "where to begin" and "what to answer" on your rounds, and will probably avoid many a dressing down from your superiors. I now offer to you a resource that I wish had been available to me. Good luck!

# Acknowledgments

I thank my wife, Wendy, for giving me the support, patience, and encouragement throughout this process, and for putting up with me sitting on the couch with my laptop every day. I also thank my mother, father, and brother, who have always supported everything I have done. I am also thankful for the faculty, residents, and nursing staff at the University of South Florida and Tampa General Hospital, for supporting me throughout my residency, and not laughing at me when I did not know the correct answer.

I would also like to specifically thank the following people, who contributed to the completion of this book:

**Darren J. DePalma, M.D.**
Resident Physician, USF Emergency Medicine Residency
Tampa, FL

**Charlotte Derr, M.D., R.D.M.S., F.A.C.E.P.**
Assistant Program Director, USF Emergency
    Medicine Residency
Tampa, FL

**Kelly P. O'Keefe, M.D., F.A.C.E.P.**
Program Director, USF Emergency Medicine Residency
Medical Director, Tampa General Hospital
    Adult Emergency Care Center
Tampa, FL

**Richard Paula, M.D., F.A.C.E.P., F.A.A.E.M.**
Director of Research
Assistant Professor, USF Emergency Medicine Residency
Tampa, FL

**Adriana Paula Suarez, M.D., F.A.C.O.G.**
Attending OB/GYN, St Joseph Women's Hospital
Tampa, FL

# Contents

# Introduction

## Initial Evaluation of the Patient

The evaluation of a patient begins as soon as you pick up the chart. Read the nurse's note thoroughly (but quickly) and take note of the chief complaint; history of the present illness as presented to the nurse; past medical history; medications; allergies; social history; tetanus immunization status; LMP; and most important, vital signs. If a vital sign is abnormal, make note of it and be sure to address it. If it is missing, ask the nurse to reassess it (and document it) and also to make sure to inform you if it is abnormal. Better yet, do this yourself. This will endear yourself to the busy nurse, who will return the favor by helping you in the future. Look at items such as the pain scale, and note the character of the symptoms. If there is a discrepancy between what you have been told and what the nurse has written, identify and explain it, verifying the data with the patient. Patients appreciate not having to tell the same story several times, so whatever you can learn ahead of time is appreciated; the patients will be happier, and you will look better.

When you walk into the room, begin to observe everything you can about the patient while you walk over and introduce yourself. If the patient is in distress, it is perfectly acceptable to introduce yourself and immediately assess the airway patency, listen to the lungs, and check the pulse. Once you have established that the patient is not going to "code" in front of you, be sure to give your full name and title.

Some students prefer "medical student," whereas others prefer "student physician." Either way, it is important that all health care workers identify themselves and their positions. Some patients will refer to you as "doctor"; be aware that some authorities say that you should correct the patient.

Classically, during the physical examination, the medical student or physician should stand/sit on the patient's *right* side. It is fine to perform the examination while you are questioning the patient. Be complete, both in the questioning and in the examination. It is far better to conduct the H&P in an all-inclusive fashion, obtaining valuable information in the process, than it is to take a "shotgun" approach with the laboratory tests and radiology examinations. With an H&P, you can better assess the patient and direct the workup, saving time and money, and satisfying everyone more as the patient moves through the medical system with greater speed. For example, if the patient complains of having "passed out" two or three times, take the time to gather important details about the circumstances surrounding the syncopal episode. Differentiate between lightheadedness/orthostasis and vertigo when the patient states that he or she is "dizzy." Assess the patient's orientation and mental status early, so you have a better idea of the reliability of the information provided. Take the time to watch the patient walk or go to radiology or down the hall to the bathroom.

Much information can be gleaned from the patient without asking the patient questions. Consider the following:

- Is the patient dyspneic (may not be able to give history due to condition or may require treatment before giving full history)?
- Is the patient in the "tripod" position (asthma)?
- Does the patient have an open soda can/fast-food bag on the tray (indicating good appetite)?

■ Is the patient's significant other hovering around, answering all questions for the patient (possible abuse)?

■ What IV drips does the patient have (provides information about patient's current condition)?

■ Is the patient pressing the PCA button constantly (uncontrolled pain)?

Initially, it is best to ask open-ended questions such as the following:

■ How do you feel this morning?

■ What brought you into the clinic/hospital this morning?

Let the patient tell his or her own "story" before interrupting, but do not allow him or her to control the interview.

Be sure to end the conversation politely. If you promise the patient juice or more pain medication, make sure your directions are carried out; the patient will not forget. Also ask the patient and family members if they have any questions. Poor patient rapport has been shown to be a factor in whether a patient pursues litigation.

## Presenting the Patient

Presenting to residents and attending physicians may be the most important (and at times nerve-racking) task you face as a medical student. But with practice and clear, concise, and honest communication, you will begin to feel comfortable presenting the patients whom you have evaluated. One thing to keep in mind is to understand the setting in which you find yourself. Presenting a patient to an attending physician in the emergency department is vastly different from presenting to an internist, a general surgeon, or an Ob/Gyn. This discussion is a general guide medical students should follow when presenting to any upper-level or resident physicians. Keep in mind, however, that some specialties require more detail about certain topics (e.g., Ob/Gyn and pregnancy history) than others.

Present the history and physical examination in an organized fashion, making it to the point, but not so brief that you omit critical information. Tailor your physical examination, reporting those pertinent positives and negatives that allow you to assess a problem adequately and rule out other significant issues. Make sure that your superiors know that you have completed a comprehensive examination and history, but do not discuss nonpertinent matters unless specifically asked to do so.

For example, start with a general statement: "Mr. Smith is a 38-year-old male with a history of X, Y, and Z who was admitted for (chief complaint/diagnosis)." Depending on the situation (e.g., first presentation of the first hospital stay, third hospital stay), present the pertinent positives and negatives (e.g., chest pain resolved, no pain at catheterization site). Be sure to note current "hospital day," "postop day," "central venous catheter day," or "antibiotic day."

Next, present the current vital signs and perhaps the vital signs of the night before ($T_{current}$ is 99.5°F; $T_{max}$ last night was 102.4°F). Do not forget input/outputs (especially NG tube, Foley), daily weights, or the last bowel movement. Pertinent physical examination findings should be next (e.g., no erythema around incision site, absent bowel sounds). Some residents/attendings expect you to know the medications that the patient is currently taking as well as the current "antibiotic day." Your assessment should include all of the conditions for which the patient is currently being treated (pneumonia, renal failure, DVT prophylaxis). If the pneumonia is resolving clinically, be sure to say so.

When you are through relating your findings, do not stop—this is the classic medical student error. Make a clear and precise summary, identify the items you need to address, discuss the differential diagnosis, and identify the orders for testing and treatment that you think should be initiated. As a medical student, you should have a good idea of the "plan" for the patient. If you can switch the patient to oral medicines, or believe the patient is ready for discharge home, present this information now.

The most important concepts to bear in my mind about making a presentation are the following:

1. Each resident or attending physician prefers a particular style of presentation that you will have to learn.
2. You will probably present incorrect information at some point. As a medical student, it is your responsibility to know "everything" (or almost everything) about your patient. However, sometimes a resident or attending does not want to know "everything," that is why you should get an idea of the type of presentation that your superiors prefer. Also, by including alternate diagnoses or a differential diagnosis that has not been previously mentioned, you may stimulate some teaching or even discover something that you missed. Above all, presenting is a learning experience.
3. Be available to the resident and attending without being a nuisance. If you wander off, you will never get to present. Follow up on results and perform repeat assessments of the patient, notifying your physician when the chance is available. Find opportunities to present the patient to the consultant and ask for feedback to determine if he or she understood what you were trying to convey.

Always stay involved: do the menial tasks for the resident, the patient, and the nurse, and you will be given many more opportunities to perform the big jobs. When you have finished presenting, and your attendings/residents have discussed the plan, pay close attention (take notes if you need to), and make sure that everything that was discussed is completed during the day (e.g., NG tube is removed, CXR is checked, patient is tolerating diet, antibiotic sensitivities are congruent with current treatment, consultants' plan is clear). One last piece of advice: the medical student who is anxious to "get the work done and go home" is spotted easily and may be interpreted as an uninterested student who does not care very much for the current rotation. By giving 100% of your energy, you will be viewed as an important part of the team, learn more, experience more, hopefully get a good review on your evaluation, and perhaps even receive a strong letter of recommendation should the time come.

## Laboratory Studies to Order

Determination of values is complicated by sex, age, clinical condition (e.g., septic, stress, pain), diet, malnutrition, drugs, time of day, and position of the patient when the specimen is drawn. Normal laboratory values are the mean values in a healthy population ± two standard deviations, which includes about 95% of the population. For interpretation of blood chemistries, see Table 1-1. For interpretation of CBC results, see Table 1-2.

## TABLE 1-1

### Blood Chemistry Interpretation

| Test | Increased in | Decreased in |
|------|-------------|--------------|
| Albumin | Dehydration | Malnutrition, nephrosis, liver failure, burns, metastatic cancer |
| Alkaline phosphatase | Bone metastases, Paget disease, fractures, hyperparathyroidism | Hypoparathyroidism |
| ALT (SGPT) | Liver disease, obstructive jaundice, mononucleosis, pancreatitis, alcohol ingestion | Vitamin $B_6$ deficiency |
| Amylase | Pancreatitis, GI obstruction, mesenteric ischemia, parotitis, mumps, renal disease, postoperative abdominal surgery | |
| AST (SGOT) | Liver disease, MI, muscular dystrophy, pancreatitis, eclampsia, alcohol ingestion | Vitamin $B_6$ deficiency |
| Bilirubin | Liver disease, obstructive jaundice, hemolytic anemias | |
| Calcium | Hyperparathyroidism, bone metastases, malignancy, myeloma, sarcoidosis, hypervitaminosis D | Hypoparathyroidism, renal failure, pancreatitis, vitamin D deficiency |
| CPK | MI, rhabdomyolysis, burns, status epilepticus | |
| Creatinine | Renal failure, dehydration, diet, muscle disease | Aging |

*(Continued)*

## TABLE 1-1

### Blood Chemistry Interpretation (*continued*)

| Test | Increased in | Decreased in |
|------|-------------|-------------|
| Glucose | DM, thiazides, glucocorticoids | Excess insulin, insulinoma, liver failure, malabsorption, pancreatitis |
| LDH | MI, hemolytic anemia, leukemia, PCP pneumonia, liver disease | |
| Lipase | Pancreatitis | |
| Magnesium | Renal disease | Diarrhea, dehydration, malabsorption, malnutrition |
| Phosphorous | Renal failure, hypoparathyroidism, lactic acidosis, cell lysis, leukemia | Hyperparathyroidism, cirrhosis, hypokalemia, alcoholism, gout |
| Potassium | Hyperkalemic acidosis, adrenal insufficiency, hemolysis, ACE inhibitors | Cirrhosis, malnutrition, vomiting/diarrhea, insulin administration |
| Sodium | Dehydration, diabetes insipidus, excess salt ingestion, diuresis | Excess ADH, vomiting/diarrhea, heart failure, diuretics, adrenal insufficiency |
| TSH | Hypothyroidism, amiodarone | Hyperthyroidism, thyroid dose excess, corticosteroids, phenytoin |
| Total protein | Multiple myeloma, sarcoidosis, SLE, dehydration | Burns, cirrhosis, overhydration |
| BUN | Renal disease, dehydration, GI bleeding, shock, MI | Liver failure, overhydration, pregnancy |
| Uric acid | Gout, renal failure, diuretics, leukemia, hemolytic anemia | Uricosuric drugs, allopurinol |

### TABLE 1-2

## Complete Blood Count Interpretation

| Test | Increased in | Decreased in |
|---|---|---|
| Eosinophils | Parasites, asthma | |
| Hgb | Polycythemia vera, dehydration, burns, COPD, CHF | Blood loss, bone marrow suppression, hemoglobinopathies, iron deficiency anemia, pregnancy |
| MCV | Pernicious anemia, folic acid deficiency, alcohol abuse | Iron deficiency anemia, lead poisoning, thalassemia |
| Platelet count | Dehydration, acute inflammatory process | DIC, ITP, TTP, aspirin, splenomegaly, chemotherapy, liver disease, leukemia |
| Polymorphonuclear neutrophils | Acute bacterial infection, stress, inflammatory processes, tissue necrosis, leukemia | Hepatitis, influenza, typhoid fever, mumps, bone marrow depletion, antineoplastic drugs, lithium |
| RBC | High altitudes, smokers, polycythemia vera, hypoxia | Anemia, acute hemorrhage, bone marrow suppression |
| Reticulocyte count | Sickle cell anemia, recent blood loss | Cirrhosis, folic acid deficiency, bone marrow suppression |

# 2 Respiratory System

## Asthma

Asthma is a chronic inflammatory disorder secondary to three components: airway inflammation, intermittent airflow obstruction, and bronchial hyperresponsiveness. Patients experience recurrent episodes of wheezing, chest tightness, and coughing. These episodes are usually reversible and improve within minutes to hours with treatment. A decreased $FEV_1/FVC$ ratio classically reverses with bronchodilators.

### Pertinent Positives/Negatives: OPQRST

- **O**nset: previous history of asthma and/or COPD or first episode of dyspnea, length of time since the current episode began, medication compliance
- **P**rovocative/**P**alliative: worsens with exercise, environmental allergens, smoking; triggered by infections
- **Q**uality: intubation if required, ICU admissions for asthma, number of emergency department visits, number of albuterol doses used per day, best spirometry measures
- **R**egion/**R**adiation: not applicable
- **S**everity: 1 to 10
- **T**iming: constant or intermittent

Associated features: coughing, wheezing, dyspnea, fever, sputum production, drug use, foreign body aspiration, steroid use, URI symptoms, stress, allergens

**Physical Examination**

■ Fever, tachycardia, tachypnea, wheezing (may not be present in severe cases), accessory muscle use, AMS, increased PA chest diameter, pulsus paradoxus, hyperresonance to percussion, decreased breath sounds, prolonged expiratory duration

■ Spirometry results (mild asthma >80% PEFR/$FEV_1$, severe asthma <60% PEFR/$FEV_1$)

 **Laboratory Studies**

■ CXR, PFTs (PEFR)

■ Consider ABG, ECG, CBC (eosinophilia)

 **Management**

■ ABCs, $O_2$, $beta_2$ agonists, steroids, ipratropium

■ Consider magnesium sulfate, epinephrine, leukotriene inhibitors, CPAP, intubation, ketamine

✖ **Pearls**

■ "Not all that wheezes is asthma" (do not forget bronchiolitis, foreign body, CF)

■ Atopic triad: wheezing, eczema, seasonal rhinitis

■ Other conditions that can mimic asthma: CHF, upper airway obstruction, foreign body, carcinoma, vocal cord dysfunction

■ Increasing $Pco_2$ (from low or normal) on ABG may indicate patient fatigue and looming respiratory failure.

---

## Chronic Obstructive Pulmonary Disease (COPD)

COPD is a chronic disease characterized by airflow limitation that is not fully reversible. Asthma, chronic bronchitis (productive cough lasting at least 3 months per year for 2 years), and emphysema (terminal airway destruction) are part of COPD. In this condition, the $FEV_1$/FEV ratio is less than normal (<0.75). COPD is the fourth most common cause of death in the United States.

## Pertinent Positives/Negatives: OPQRST

- **O**nset: history of chronic bronchitis/emphysema
- **P**rovocative/**P**alliative: worsens with smoking, occupational/ allergen exposure, medication noncompliance; may improve with oxygen, or albuterol and/or ipratropium treatments
- **Q**uality: number of albuterol and/or ipratropium treatments per day, required intubation in the past, when and what antibiotics last used
- **R**egion/**R**adiation: not applicable
- **S**everity: 1 to 10
- **T**iming: constant or intermittent symptoms

Associated features: cough (minimal vs. productive sputum), dyspnea, chest discomfort, recurrent "bronchitis" or upper respiratory infections, hemoptysis, smoking, edema, weight gain or loss, family history, overweight, heart failure, cyanosis, somnolence, fevers, oxygen dependence, tremor, confusion

##  Physical Examination

- Fever, tachypnea, tachycardia
- Obesity or cachexia
- Decreased breath sounds, wheezing, rhonchi or crackles, cyanosis, pursed lip breathing, prolonged expiratory phase, increased AP diameter (barrel chest), distant heart sounds, cough, lower extremity erythema or edema, JVD, accessory muscle use

## 🔬 Laboratory Studies (Fig. 2-1)

■ CBC, BMP, CXR, PFTs (PEFR)

■ Consider ABG, ECG, BNP

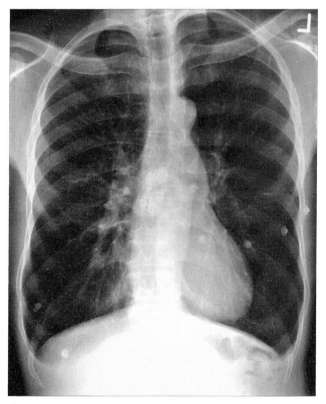

**Figure 2-1** Chest radiograph showing classic findings of COPD. Note the hyperinflation, paucity of lung markings, flattened diaphragms, hyperlucency of lung fields, and the lower ribs seen above the diaphragm. (*Courtesy of Brigham and Women's Hospital, Boston, Massachusetts.*)

## 🔖 Management

- ABCs, $O_2$, beta$_2$ agonists, steroids, antibiotics, ipratropium
- Consider CPAP or BIPAP, intubation, smoking cessation, theophylline, pneumococcal and/or influenza vaccines, long-term oxygen therapy when $O_2$ saturation <90% on room air (or $PaO_2$ <60 mm Hg).

## ✳️ Pearls

- "Pink Puffer": emphysema, decreased breath sounds, dyspnea, hypercarbia or hypoxia, barrel chest, thin
- "Blue Bloater": chronic bronchitis, rhonchi, productive cough, mild dyspnea, overweight, edematous
- Be aware of "$CO_2$ retainers" who may deteriorate slowly with supplemental $O_2$ (increases their $PCO_2$ due to loss of hypoxemic drive).
- Only two treatments have been shown to improve COPD: smoking cessation and supplemental $O_2$.
- Be aware of alpha-1 antitrypsin deficiency, an inheritable form of emphysema in a young patient with a minimal history of smoking.

## Dyspnea

Dyspnea is a subjective feeling of difficult or uncomfortable breathing or "shortness of breath." The differential diagnosis should include COPD, CHF, pneumonia, PE, pneumothorax, foreign body obstruction, pulmonary edema, pleural effusion, ischemic heart disease, unstable angina, MI, angioedema, myasthenia gravis, Guillain-Barré syndrome, and anaphylactic reaction. Other conditions that should be ruled out include lung mass, influenza, bronchitis, epiglottitis, hyperventilation, pericarditis, anemia, and psychogenic/panic attack/anxiety.

### Pertinent Positives/Negatives: OPQRST

■ **O**nset: time of initiation (sudden or insidious [subtle]): after trauma, possible medication noncompliance

■ **P**rovocative/**P**alliative: worsens with activity or exercise, lying flat or sleeping, environmental triggers; improves with sitting up, being exposed to cold air

■ **Q**uality: not applicable

■ **R**egion/**R**adiation: chest, back, abdominal pain; similar episodes of same dyspnea

■ **S**everity: 1 to 10

■ **T**iming: constant or intermittent

Associated features: insomnia (waking several times per night), increasing number of pillows, fever, cough (productive), color of sputum, generalized muscle weakness, smoking, audible wheezing

 **Physical Examination**

■ Determine severity with initial assessment

■ Findings include fever, tachypnea, tachycardia, accessory muscle use, stridor, "conversational dyspnea," breathlessness, agitation, AMS, paradoxical abdominal wall movement, $S_3$ or $S_4$, JVD, deviated trachea, asymmetric expansion of chest, pleural friction rub, decreased breath sounds, cyanosis, hypotension, RUQ pain, consolidation, wheezing/rhonchi/crackles, chest wall tenderness, lower extremity erythema/edema/tenderness, upper airway swelling, and facial swelling

## 🔬 Laboratory Studies

- Pulse oximetry, ECG, CXR
- Consider ABG, PEFR, cardiac enzymes, BNP, D-dimer, Doppler U/S, x-ray of soft tissue of neck

## 💊 Management

- Treat underlying disorder
- Correct hypoxia, hypovolemia

## ✳️ Pearls

- "Not all that wheezes is asthma."
- Life-threatening causes of dyspnea: upper airway obstruction, MI, pneumothorax, myasthenia gravis, asthma, angioedema, anaphylaxis, PE
- Tracheal deviation and JVD are **very late** signs of tension pneumothorax.
- Crackles ("crushing of fine leaves or rubbing of Velcro") are usually diagnostic of interstitial edema (pneumonia, CHF).
- Rhonchi ("snoring or cooing of a wood pigeon") are usually secretions.
- A localized, persistent rhonchus or wheeze is cancer until proven otherwise.
- Differential diagnosis of dyspnea:
  - **3As:** three airways: **A**irway obstruction, **A**naphylaxis, **A**sthma
  - **3Ps:** three pulmonaries: **P**neumothorax, **PE**, **P**ulmonary edema
  - **3Cs:** three cardiacs: **C**ardiogenic pulmonary edema, **C**ardiac ischemia, **C**ardiac tamponade
  - **3Ms:** three metabolics: (**DOC**) **D**KA, **O**rganophosphates, **C**arbon monoxide poisoning

## Hemoptysis

Hemoptysis is the coughing up of blood from the respiratory tract. The condition can be benign or life-threatening.

### Pertinent Positives/Negatives: OPQRST

- **O**nset: length of time symptoms have been present
- **P**rovocative/**P**alliative: may worsen with continued coughing
- **Q**uality: back, shoulder, chest, or abdominal pain
- **R**egion/**R**adiation: not applicable
- **S**everity: 1 to 10
- **T**iming: constant or intermittent

Associated features: fevers, chills, recent URI, productive cough (color of sputum), weight loss, nausea and/or vomiting, dyspnea, foreign body ingestion, recent trauma, abrupt onset of cough, syncope, orthostatic symptoms, symptoms of PE

#### Hemoptysis: CAVITATES

**C**HF
**A**irway disease, bronchiectasis
**V**asculitis/**V**ascular malformations
**I**nfection (e.g., TB)
**T**rauma
**A**nticoagulation
**T**umor
**E**mbolism
**S**tomach

 **Physical Examination**

- Fever, tachypnea, tachycardia, hypotension, orthostatic vital signs

- Pallor; nasal, facial, or pharyngeal hemorrhage; crackles or rhonchi; lymphadenopathy; clubbing; evidence of liver disease; pale conjunctiva; evidence of IV drug use

## Laboratory Studies

- Pulse oximetry, CBC, PT/PTT/INR, CMP, CXR, type and cross for PRBCs
- Consider bronchoscopy, CT, D-dimer, PPD, ABG, sputum stains and cytology

## Management

- ABCs, hemostasis, consider ETT
- Treat underlying disorder
- Lie the patient on side of bleeding to avoid transfer of hemorrhage to unaffected side.

## Pearls

- For massive hemoptysis, think of bronchiectasis and neoplasms.
- Differential diagnosis of hemoptysis:
    - Infections: pneumonia, tuberculosis, bronchitis, aspergillosis, lung abscesses, parasitic diseases
    - Cardiovascular: PE, CHF, pulmonary hypertension, mitral stenosis, aortic aneurysm, pulmonary malformations
    - Iatrogenic: bronchoscopy, heart catheterization, bronchial biopsy
    - Malignancies
    - Trauma
    - Foreign body aspiration
    - Hematologic: platelet dysfunction, coagulopathy, anticoagulant therapy

## Lung Cancer

Lung cancer is the leading cause of cancer death in the US in both males and females. The 5-year survival rate is less than 20%. Lung cancer can be divided into small cell lung cancer and non–small cell lung cancer. Patients may be asymptomatic, or they may present with a change in chronic cough, hemoptysis, pneumonia, and/or weight loss.

### Pertinent Positives/Negatives: OPQRST

■ **O**nset: length of time symptoms have been present
■ **P**rovocative/**P**alliative: not applicable
■ **Q**uality: chest, back, or abdominal pain; headaches
■ **R**egion/**R**adiation: not applicable
■ **S**everity: 1 to 10
■ **T**iming: constant or intermittent

Associated features: smoking; asbestos exposure; history of COPD; cough; hemoptysis; recurrent pneumonia; wheezing; postprandial coughing; stridor; arm weakness or paresthesias; weight loss; cachexia; night sweats; diarrhea; sweating; flushing; dyspnea; bone pain; new-onset headaches, seizures, or visual changes

### Physical Examination

■ Often unremarkable
■ Cachexia, fever, stridor, wheezing, atelectasis, crackles, cyanosis, JVD, lymphadenopathy, clubbing

### Laboratory Studies

■ CBC, CMP (hypercalcemia), CXR, pulse oximetry, ECG
■ Consider ABG, CT, sputum cytology, bronchoscopy

**Management**

- ABCs
- Surgical resection, chemotherapy

### Pearls

- As many as one fourth of all patients are asymptomatic at diagnosis.
- Cushing syndrome: production of ACTH by small cell carcinoma
- As many as 80% of lung cancers occur in smokers or former smokers.
- Adenocarcinoma is the most frequent type of lung cancer, with squamous cell carcinoma second.
- Pancoast tumor (apical tumor): upper extremity pain, hand muscle atrophy, Horner syndrome (unilateral ptosis, miosis, anhidrosis)
- SVC syndrome: compression of the SVC with impaired venous drainage (dilated neck veins, upper extremity or facial edema)
- Eaton Lambert syndrome: myasthenia gravis–like disease, but muscles become stronger with repetitive use; due to lung cancer

## Pleural Effusion

Pleural effusion is the abnormal accumulation of fluid in the pleural space. Abnormal permeability of pleural membranes, change in oncotic pressure, increased hydrostatic pressures, and infection are some mechanisms for fluid accumulation. Pleural effusions are categorized by exudative or transudative. Patients may be asymptomatic.

## Pertinent Positives/Negatives: OPQRST

■ **O**nset: length of time symptoms have been present
■ **P**rovocative/**P**alliative: worsens at night; improves with breathing treatments, thoracentesis
■ **Q**uality: history of "fluid in the lung"; cardiac, liver, lung, pancreas, or kidney disease; history of cancer
■ **R**egion/**R**adiation: chest, back, neck, or abdominal
■ **S**everity: 1 to 10
■ **T**iming: constant or intermittent

Associated features: cough, dyspnea, fever or chills, night sweats, weight loss or gain, trauma, edema, hemoptysis, TB, HIV, sputum production

 **Physical Examination**

Fever, diminished breath sounds, dullness to percussion, pleural friction rub, JVD, cutaneous evidence of liver disease, lymphadenopathy, $S_3$, edema, clubbing

 **Laboratory Studies**

■ CXR, CBC, CMP, ECG, pulse oximetry
■ Pleural fluid analysis: Gram stain, cytology, LDH, pH, cell count, culture, protein, glucose, amylase (Table 2-1)

### TABLE 2-1

**Diagnostic Classification of Pleural Effusion Using Pleural Fluid Analysis**

|  | Transudative | Exudative |
|---|---|---|
| LDH | <200 U/mL | LDH > two thirds of upper limit of serum LDH |
| Fluid:serum protein ratio | <0.5 | >0.5 |

## Management

- Treat underlying cause
- Symptomatic drainage/relief via thoracentesis

## Pearls

- Transudative: CHF, cirrhosis, nephritic syndrome, PE
- Exudative: infection, cancer, pancreatitis
- It takes 250–500 ml to see lateral costophrenic angle blunting on upright CXR.
- A pleural effusion is best detected on a lateral decubitus CXR.
- Bloody effusion: malignancy
- Yellow effusion: empyema
- Putrid odor: anaerobic infection

---

## Pneumonia

Pneumonia is infection of the alveolar portions of the lung with inflammatory exudates. Pneumonia developing outside the hospital is considered **community-acquired**, whereas pneumonia developing as an inpatient is considered **nosocomial** or **hospital-acquired**. Pneumonia is the sixth leading cause of death. The classic presentation is cough, sputum production, dyspnea, fevers, and pleuritic chest pain. Clinicians should be aware of atypical pneumonia; patients can present with headaches and GI symptoms.

### Risk Factors for Pneumonia: INSPIRATION

**I**mmunosuppression
**N**eoplasia
**S**ecretion retention
**P**ulmonary edema

**I**mpaired alveolar macrophages
**R**espiratory tract infection (prior)
**A**ntibiotics and cytotoxics
**T**racheal instrumentation
**IV** drug abuse
**O**ther (general debility, immobility)
**N**eurologic impairment of cough reflex (e.g., neuromuscular junction disorders)

## Pertinent Positives/Negatives: OPQRST

■ **O**nset: time that symptoms began
■ **P**rovocative/**P**alliative: worsens with antipyretics, antibiotics, albuterol treatments
■ **Q**uality: not applicable
■ **R**egion/**R**adiation: chest pain, RUQ and/or LUQ abdominal pain (especially in pediatrics), lower extremity erythema or edema, headaches, GI symptoms (diarrhea in *Legionella* pneumonia)
■ **S**everity: 1 to 10
■ **T**iming: constant or intermittent symptoms

Associated features: fever, cough, sputum (color, consistency), hemoptysis, night sweats, dyspnea (exertional vs. constant), smoking, alcohol use, home situation (nursing home, jail, homeless), HIV, TB exposure, solid organ transplant, splenectomy, malaise, nausea and vomiting, AMS, rigors or chills, occupation, environmental exposure (Southwest US, spelunking, poultry)

### Physical Examination

■ Fever, tachypnea, tachycardia, hypotension, decreased breath sounds, rhonchi, crackles, consolidation, wheezing, egophony, tactile fremitus, pleural rub, AMS, diaphoresis

- Evidence of DVT, poor dentition, evidence of aspiration, other source of infection

## Laboratory Studies

- CBC, CMP, CXR, sputum examination
- Consider ABG, blood cultures, ECG, CD4, *Legionella* urine antigen, culture and Gram stain

## Management

- Consider IV antibiotics (ceftriaxone/azithromycin vs. Levofloxacin), admission
- Treat empirically or for suspected pathogen

## Pearls (Table 2-2)

- Adequate sputum specimen must have <10 squamous cells, >25 WBCs
- *Streptococcus pneumoniae* is the most common cause of CAP.
- "Currant jelly" sputum: *Klebsiella*, aspiration, alcoholics
- Be aware of hyponatremia and *Legionella*.
- Exposure to bird droppings: *Chlamydia psittaci* or *Histoplasma*
- CF: *Pseudomonas* species
- Immigrants: TB
- In HIV-positive patients, be aware of the following factors: *Pneumocystis carinii* pneumonia, low CD4 count, not taking HIV medications, increased LDH, diffuse bilateral infiltrates on CXR.
- Postinfluenza pneumonia: *Staphylococcus aureus*

**TABLE 2-2**

Characteristics of "Classic" Pneumonia Syndromes

| Organism | H&P | Sputum Gram Stain | CXR | Therapy |
|---|---|---|---|---|
| *Haemophilus influenzae* | Smoking, COPD | Encapsulated gram-negative rods | Lobar consolidation | PCN, macrolide, cephalosporin |
| *Klebsiella pneumoniae* | Alcoholism, COPD | Encapsulated gram-negative rods | Lobar consolidation | Aminoglycoside, cefazolin |
| *Legionella pneumophila* | Cooling systems, COPD, alcoholism | Gram-negative rods | Bilateral patchy | Erythromycin, rifampin |
| *Mycoplasma pneumoniae* | Young, healthy | No organisms | Bilateral interstitial infiltrates | Erythromycin, tetracycline |

(*Continued*)

## TABLE 2-2

### Characteristics of "Classic" Pneumonia Syndromes (continued)

| Organism | H&P | Sputum Gram Stain | CXR | Therapy |
|----------|-----|-------------------|-----|---------|
| *Pneumocystis carinii* | HIV infection | Cysts on methenamine silver stain | Perihilar "batwing" infiltrates | Trimethoprim/sulfamethoxazole or pentamidine |
| *Pseudomonas aeruginosa* | Nursing home | Gram-negative rods | Patchy lower lung consolidations | Aminoglycoside, cefazolin |
| *Staphylococcus aureus* | Postinfluenza virus, IV drug use | Gram-positive cocci in clusters | Lobar construction or cavitary | PCN, vancomycin |
| *Streptococcus pneumoniae* | Extreme of age, rusty sputum | Lancet-shaped gram-positive diplococci | Lobar consolidation | PCN, macrolide, FQ |

PCN: penicillin; FQ: fluoroquinolone

(From Mick N, et al., *Blueprints Emergency Medicine, 2nd ed*. Malden, MA: Blackwell Publishing, 2006.)

## Pneumothorax

Pneumothorax is a potentially fatal condition that occurs when air enters the pleural space spontaneously or due to trauma. Spontaneous pneumothorax occurs usually in tall, thin males who smoke. Traumatic pneumothorax develops when the chest wall or pulmonary tissue acts as a one-way valve, allowing air to enter into the pleural space and trapping the air during expiration. Tension pneumothorax can be life-threatening by progressively collapsing the lung, causing a mediastinal shift and impairing cardiac output.

### Pertinent Positives/Negatives: **OPQRST**

■ **O**nset: possible sudden onset or association with trauma, coughing, cocaine use (Valsalva maneuver after inhaling to increase effect of drug)

■ **P**rovocative/**P**alliative: worsens with deep breath, coughing, rest, lying flat

■ **Q**uality: pleuritic chest pain, history of collapsed lung, recent SCUBA

■ **R**egion/**R**adiation: chest, shoulder, back, neck or face, or abdominal pain

■ **S**everity: 1 to 10

■ **T**iming: constant or intermittent

Associated features: dyspnea, history of COPD, smoking, marfanoid or history of Marfan syndrome, hemoptysis, menses (catamenial pneumothorax), recent instrumentation (surgery, central lines)

###  Physical Examination

■ Tachypnea, tachycardia, hypoxia, hypotension

■ Decreased breath sounds, asymmetric expansion of chest, JVD, mediastinal shift, hyperresonance, flail chest, deviated trachea, crepitus, subcutaneous emphysema, height-to-weight ratio, marfanoidism

### 🔬 Laboratory Studies

■ CXR
■ Consider expiratory films, chest CT, ABG

### 💊 Management

■ $O_2$
■ Small pneumothoraces can resolve spontaneously; observe with serial CXRs.
■ If considering tension pneumothorax, use immediate needle decompression followed by chest tube placement.

### ✳ Pearls

■ A tension pneumothorax is a **clinical** diagnosis, not a radiographic one.
■ Needle decompression: large-bore angiocatheter/needle over the second intercostal space, midclavicular line, superior to rib on the affected side

## Pulmonary Embolus (PE)

PE is a potentially fatal complication of venous thrombosis migrated into pulmonary vasculature, resulting in occlusion. Evaluation for PE should be started if the diagnosis of PE is suspected. PE leads to hypoxemia, pulmonary infarction, and right-sided heart failure. The third most common cause of death in the United States, PE is likely the second leading cause of unexpected death. Approximately 90% of DVTs that embolize at the lungs are from the lower extremities.

### Pertinent Positives/Negatives: OPQRST

■ **O**nset: sudden or insidious

■ **P**rovocative/**P**alliative: not applicable

■ **Q**uality: associated with pain or only dyspnea and/or hemoptysis

■ **R**egion/**R**adiation: chest pain (qualify and quantify), back pain, chest wall tenderness, shoulder and RUQ/LUQ pain, extremity pain and/or swelling

■ **S**everity: 1 to 10

■ **T**iming: constant or intermittent symptoms

Associated features: difficult and/or painful respiration, wheezing, palpitations, syncope, hemoptysis, nausea and/or vomiting, recent bed rest, recent surgery, history of DVT or PE, recent pregnancy, smoking, oral contraceptives, recent hospitalization, long-distance travel, recent trauma, dizziness or weakness, recent fracture, active or history of cancer, coagulopathies (protein C or S deficiencies), family history of blood clots, vaginal delivery (amniotic fluid embolus)

###  Physical Examination

■ Fever, tachycardia, hypertension or hypotension, AMS, respiratory distress, diaphoresis, cyanosis, anxiety, JVD, facial swelling or erythema, crackles, rhonchi, wheeze (isolated), pleural friction rub, $S_3$, $S_4$, accentuated $S_2$, heart murmur, reproducible chest tenderness, lower extremity edema or erythema, soft compartments of lower extremities, evidence of thrombophlebitis

■ Presence of central venous catheter

### 🔬 Laboratory Studies
- Pulse oximetry, D-dimer, ECG, CXR
- Consider ABG, lower extremity U/S, V/Q scan, chest CT, pulmonary angiogram

### 💊 Management
- ABCs, heparin plus warfarin; consider TPA, surgery (thrombectomy)
- Correct hypoxemia
- Consider IVC filter

### ✳️ Pearls
- Virchow angle: hypercoagulability, stasis, venous injury
- If survivors of PE are untreated, one third will die of future embolism.
- Hampton hump (wedge-shaped infarct) and Westermark sign (oligemia) are rare on CXR. Be aware of cardiomegaly and basilar atelectasis; however, a normal CXR may be present in 25% of cases.
- Most common ECG findings: sinus tachycardia or inverted T waves in $V_1$-$V_3$. Be aware of "S1Q3T3," RVH, and RBBB.
- Patients with PE can have intermittent shortness of breath.
- As many as 13% of patients with acute PE develop syncope.
- The "classic" triad of PE (dyspnea, pleuritic chest pain, hemoptysis) is uncommon.

---

## Sarcoidosis

---

Sarcoidosis is a systemic disease of noncaseating epithelioid granulomas that can affect any organ system, but usually involves the lungs. The cause of sarcoidosis is unknown.

In the United States, sarcoidosis is most common in black females. Its clinical presentation is variable, and it is often discovered incidentally on routine CXR.

### Pertinent Positives/Negatives
Associated features: fever, weight loss, fatigue, cough, malaise, arthritis, shin discoloration/sensitivity

 ### Physical Examination
■ Palpable lymph nodes, erythema nodosum, plaques/nodules, scar discoloration

 ### Laboratory Studies
■ CBC, CXR (bilateral hilar lymphadenopathy), serum ACE levels, CMP (hypercalcemia)
■ Consider PFT, bronchoscopic biopsy

### Management
■ Steroids

---

## Tuberculosis (TB)

---

TB is an infection caused by *Mycobacterium tuberculosis*. TB may involve multiple organ systems but usually remains confined to the lung. The majority of cases of symptomatic TB are actually due to reactivation of old infection. Transmission is by aerosolized droplets.

### Pertinent Positives/Negatives: OPQRST
■ **O**nset: length of time symptoms have been present
■ **P**rovocative/**P**alliative: possible recurrence of symptoms after previous antibiotics, possible medication noncompliance

- **Q**uality: history of TB, exposure to TB, previous positive PPD test, history of TB immunization
- **R**egion/**R**adiation: chest, back, or neck pain; rashes
- **S**everity: 1 to 10
- **T**iming: constant or intermittent

Associated features: immigration, immunosuppression, alcoholism, incarceration, homelessness, family member with TB, HIV, illicit drug use, cough, night sweats, fever or chills, weight loss, hemoptysis, anorexia, malaise, hematuria

## Physical Examination

- Fever, productive cough, sputum, reproducible chest pain
- Hepatosplenomegaly, lymphadenopathy, rhonchi, consolidation, AMS, friction rub

## Laboratory Studies

- CXR (cavitary lesions in upper lobe, hilar adenopathy, pleural effusions, nodules), CBC, CMP (check liver function), PPD, blood culture, sputum samples (stained for AFB)
- Consider thoracentesis (if pleural effusion)

## Management

- Treat with INH (give supplemental vitamin $B_6$), rifampin, pyrazinamide, ethambutol
- Respiratory isolation, treat contacts

## Pearls

- As many as 15% of TB cases are extrapulmonary.

■ Immunocompromised patients may not elicit a positive PPD; therefore use a control.

■ "Sterile pyuria" = TB.

### 📖 Literature

■ Alberts C, van der Mark TW, Jansen HM. *Eur Respir J.* 1995 May;8(5):682–688. Inhaled budesonide in pulmonary sarcoidosis: a double-blind, placebo-controlled study. Dutch Study Group on Pulmonary Sarcoidosis. This article reported that inhaled steroids are helpful in improving lung function in pulmonary sarcoidosis.

■ Branca P, Rodriguez RM, Rogers JT, et al. Routine measurement of pleural fluid amylase is not indicated. *Arch Intern Med.* 2001 Jan 22;161(2):228–232. The routine measurement of pleural amylase is neither clinically indicated nor cost-effective, and it should be measured only if acute pancreatitis, chronic pancreatitis, or esophageal rupture is suspected.

■ Brown MD, Vance SJ, Kline JA. An Emergency Department Guideline for the Diagnosis of Pulmonary Embolism: An Outcome Study. *Acad Emerg Med.* 2005;12(1):20–25. In low-risk patients (younger than 70 years of age with a low clinical suspicion of PE and no unexplained hypoxemia, unilateral leg swelling, recent surgery, hemoptysis, pregnancy, or prolonged duration of symptoms), negative ELISA D-dimer has a negative predictive value of 99.9% for PE.

■ Flower CDR, Jackson JE. The role of radiology in the investigation and management of patients with hemoptysis. *Clin Radiol.* 1996;51:391–400. The authors showed that CXR is diagnostic in only approximately 50% of cases.

- Henschke CI, Yankelevitz DF. *Radiol Clin North Am*. 2000 May;38(3):487–495. CT screening for lung cancer. This review concluded that CT screening for lung cancer absolutely results in earlier diagnosis but has not yet proven to decrease mortality.

- Kennedy M, Bates DW, Wright SB, et al. Do emergency department blood cultures change practice in patients with pneumonia? *Ann Emerg Med*. 2005 Nov;46(5):393–400. The authors determined that blood cultures rarely altered therapy of patients presenting to the emergency department with CAP.

- Kim S, Emerman CL, Cydulka RK, Rowe BH, Clark S, Camargo CA; MARC Investigators. Prospective multicenter study of relapse following emergency department treatment of COPD exacerbation. *Chest*. 2004 Feb;125(2):473–481. This study showed that there is a 20% relapse rate after emergency department treatment of COPD.

- Kirkpatrick AW, Sirois M, Laupland KB, et al. Hand-held thoracic sonography for detecting post-traumatic pneumothoraces: the Extended Focused Assessment with Sonography for Trauma (EFAST). *J Trauma*. 2004 Aug;57(2):288–295. This article reported that CT is the gold standard and that U/S is as sensitive as CXR (both U/S and CXR have excellent specificity [>95%] but a lower sensitivity [approximately 50–70%]).

- Lapworth R, Tarn AC, British Thoracic Society. Clinical Science Reviews Committee of the Association for Clinical Biochemistry. Commentary on the British Thoracic Society guidelines for the investigation of unilateral pleural effusion in adults. *Ann Clin Biochem*. 2006 Jan;43(Pt 1): 17–22. This review concluded that protein measurement is the single most important aspect of pleural effusion management.

■ Millar AB, Boothroyd AE, Edwards D, et al. The role of computed tomography in the investigation of unexplained hemoptysis. *Respir Med.* 1992;86:39–44. This study showed that chest CT was very helpful; CT found a diagnosis in 50% of patients when CXR and bronchoscopy were both normal.

■ Qureshi F, Zaritsky A, Welch C, et al. Clinical efficacy of racemic albuterol versus levalbuterol for the treatment of acute pediatric asthma. *Ann Emerg Med.* 2005 Jul;46(1):29–36. Treatment with Xopenex (levalbuterol) showed no difference in pediatric patients in terms of primary outcomes (changes from baseline in clinical asthma score and the percentage of predicted forced expiratory volume in 1 second after the first, third, and fifth treatments).

■ Rowe BH, Spooner CH, Ducharme FM, et al. Corticosteroids for preventing relapse following acute exacerbations of asthma. *Cochrane Database Syst Rev.* 2001;(1):CD000195. This article revealed that a short course of corticosteroids following assessment for an acute exacerbation of asthma significantly reduced the number of asthma relapses and the decreased use of beta-agonists.

■ Schreck DM, Babin S. Comparison of racemic albuterol and levalbuterol in the treatment of acute asthma in the ED. *Am J Emerg Med.* 2005 Nov;23(7):842–847. The researchers showed that there is a difference in adults, and significantly fewer admissions were also observed (13.8% vs. 28.9%, respectively; $P = 0.021$) in the levalbuterol vs. racemic albuterol group. Treatment costs were lower with levalbuterol, mainly because of a decrease in hospital admissions.

■ Seow A, Kazerooni EA, Pernicano PG, et al. Comparison of upright inspiratory and expiratory chest radiographs for detecting pneumothoraces. *AJR Am J Roentgenol*. 1996 Feb;166(2):313–316. Researchers found that inspiratory and expiratory films were equally sensitive for pneumothorax detection; inspiratory films are recommended as the initial examination choice.

■ Singh JM, Palda VA, Stanbrook MB, et al. Corticosteroid therapy for patients with acute exacerbations of chronic obstructive pulmonary disease: a systematic review. *Arch Intern Med*. 2002 Dec 9–23;162(22):2527–2536. In a systematic review, researchers found that short courses of corticosteroids in acute exacerbations of COPD improved spirometric as well as clinical outcomes.

■ Theerthakarai R, El-Halees W, Ismail M, et al. Nonvalue of the initial microbiological studies in the management of nonsevere community-acquired pneumonia. *Chest*. 2001 Jan;119(1):181–184. Initial microbiological studies (sputum Gram stain, sputum culture, and blood cultures) had no value in management of cases of nonsevere CAP without comorbid factors.

■ Value of the ventilation/perfusion scan in acute pulmonary embolism. Results of the prospective investigation of pulmonary embolism diagnosis (PIOPED). *JAMA*. 1990 May 23–30;263(20):2753–2759. The PIOPED investigators showed that clinical assessment combined with V/Q scanning established the diagnosis or exclusion of PE in only a minority of patients.

■ Van Dyck P, Vanhoenacker FM, Van den Brande P, et al. Imaging of pulmonary tuberculosis. *Eur Radiol*. 2003 Aug;13(8):1771–1785. This study showed that the CXR appearance of TB is not classic in the elderly and immunocompromised (e.g., patients with HIV, neutropenia).

■ Wood-Baker RR, Gibson PG, Hannay M, et al. Systemic corticosteroids for acute exacerbations of chronic obstructive pulmonary disease. *The Cochrane Database of Systematic Reviews 2005.* Issue 1 Art. No.: CD001288. DOI:10.1002/14651858. The authors found that steroids decrease relapse rates.

# 3 | Cardiovascular System

## Arrhythmias/Atrial Fibrillation (AF)

AF occurs when there are multiple areas of atrial myocardium discharging and contracting, resulting in a quivering of the atrial wall. The ventricular rate is normally limited from this chaotic atrial rhythm via the refractory period of the atrioventricular node. AF occurs in almost 5% of people 69 years of age and older in the United States and can result in significant morbidity and mortality. As many as 20% of strokes can be attributed to AF. It is important to discriminate between new-onset AF and chronic AF.

### Pertinent Positives/Negatives: OPQRST

- **O**nset: sudden onset of palpitations, weakness, or chest discomfort; history of AF, cardiac arrhythmia, or irregular heart beat
- **P**rovocative/**P**alliative: worse with stress (emotion, exertion, eating)
- **Q**uality: palpitations, chest pain (describe)
- **R**egion/**R**adiation: associated with abdominal pain
- **S**everity: 1 to 10
- **T**iming: constant or intermittent ("Do you feel it now?")

Associated features: chest pain, dyspnea, palpitations, nausea, diaphoresis, syncope, medication noncompliance, history of ischemic heart disease, history of thyroid disease, history of rheumatic fever, IV drug use, alcohol use, history of PE and/or DVT, recent surgery, history of lung disease

### Causes of Atrial Fibrillation: **THE ATRIAL FIBS**

**T**hyroid
**H**ypothermia
**E**mbolism (PE)
**A**lcohol ("holiday heart")
**T**rauma (cardiac contusion)
**R**ecent surgery (post-CABG)
**I**schemia
**A**trial enlargement
**L**one or idiopathic
**F**ever, anemia, high-output states
**I**nfarct
**B**ad valves (mitral stenosis)
**S**timulants (cocaine, theophylline, amphetamine, caffeine)

## Physical Examination

■ Hemodynamic instability or stability, hypertension or hypotension, tachycardia, hypoxia, diaphoresis, distal pulses in all extremities, AMS, JVD, hepatojugular reflex, CVP, cyanosis, crackles, wheezes, rhonchi, irregular rhythm, $S_3$, evidence of murmur (new/old), displaced PMI, evidence of CHF, evidence of embolic disease

■ Neuromuscular weakness, large thyroid

## Laboratory Studies

■ ECG (P waves absent, irregularly irregular rhythm) (Fig. 3-1), CXR, CBC, CMP, PT/PTT/INR, TSH, drug screen, D-dimer

■ Consider cardiac enzymes, ABG, digoxin level, alcohol level, TTE, TEE

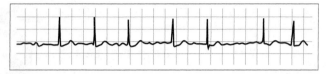

**Figure 3-1** An ECG showing the irregularly irregular pattern of atrial fibrillation. (*Reproduced by permission from Axford J. Medicine. 2nd ed. Malden, MA: Blackwell Publishing, 2004:439.*)

## Management (Table 3-1)

- Unstable
  - ABCs
  - Synchronized cardioversion and/or medication
- Stable
  - Control ventricular rate (diltiazem, beta-blocker, digoxin)
  - Antiarrhythmics and/or cardioversion
  - Evaluate cause of AF (accessory pathway)

## Pearls

- Patients with atrial fibrillation of greater than 2 days' duration should be anticoagulated for as long as 3 weeks before cardioversion.
- As many as 15% of patients in chronic AF have at least one embolic episode per year.

## Chest Pain

Chest pain is a common complaint seen in emergency departments and inpatient facilities as well as in outpatient clinics. The spectrum of diseases involving chest pain is quite broad, with very benign as well as serious life-threatening disease entities. A systematic approach to *all* patients with chest pain

## TABLE 3-1

Narrow Complex Tachycardias (QRS <0.12) with Irregular Rhythms

| Type | Atrial Rate | P-Wave Morphology | Treatment |
|------|-------------|-------------------|-----------|
| **Multifocal atrial tachycardia** | 100–200 | Varies from beat to beat (requires three or more differently shaped P waves with varying PR intervals) | • Treat underlying disorder<br>• For decompensated lung disease, treat with oxygen and bronchodilators<br>• Amiodarone, beta-blocker, or $Ca^{2+}$ channel blocker |
| **Atrial fibrillation** | 350–450 | Fibrillatory waves—no distinct P wave | • Unstable patients need emergent synchronized cardioversion<br>• Stable patients need rate control with $Ca^{2+}$ channel blocker<br>• Beta-blockers or digoxin<br>• Because of risk of intra-atrial thrombi and arterial embolism, patients with atrial fibrillation of >2 days should be anticoagulated (warfarin) first, for 3 weeks before attempts at electrical or chemical cardioversion |

(Continued)

**TABLE 3-1**

Narrow Complex Tachycardias (QRS <0.12) with Irregular Rhythms (*continued*)

| Type | Atrial Rate | P-Wave Morphology | Treatment |
|------|-------------|-------------------|-----------|
| **Wolff-Parkinson-White syndrome with atrial fibrillation** | | Fibrillatory waves—no distinct P wave | • Unstable patients need emergent synchronized cardioversion<br>• Stable patients need rate control with procainamide or amiodarone (Class I)<br>• Do not use adenosine, digoxin, $Ca^{2+}$ channel or beta-blockers as they may increase ventricular rate |

*(From Mick N, et al., Blueprints Emergency Medicine, 2nd ed. Malden, MA: Blackwell Publishing, 2006.)*

should be followed, and all immediate life-threatening events should be excluded. The differential diagnosis includes angina (stable and unstable), MI, aortic dissection, pericarditis, PE, pneumonia, pneumothorax, pleurisy, GERD, mitral valve prolapse, hypertrophic obstructive myopathy, arrhythmias, esophageal rupture, and herpes zoster. Other conditions that should be ruled out include the following:

■ Pulmonary: cough, URI, asthma/COPD, pneumomediastinum, pleural effusion

■ Gastrointestinal: GERD, esophageal foreign body, PUD, cholelithiasis

■ Musculoskeletal: rib fracture, costosternal syndrome, costochondritis (Tietze syndrome), contusion

■ Other: sickle cell disease (acute chest syndrome), cocaine abuse, pleurodynia, cocaine abuse, breast changes, connective tissue disorders

### Pericarditis: **CARDIAC RIND**

**C**ollagen vascular disease
**A**ortic aneurysm
**R**adiation
**D**rugs (hydralazine)
**I**nfections
**A**cute renal failure
**C**ardiac infarction
**R**heumatic fever
**I**njury
**N**eoplasms
**D**ressler syndrome

### Pertinent Positives/Negatives: **OPQRST**

■ **O**nset: sudden, subtle, progressive, regressive, insidious, after trauma

- **P**rovocative/**P**alliative: worsens with exertion, eating, emotion, breathing, stress (emotional or physical), movement of arms or legs; improves with NTG or positioning
- **Q**uality: sharp, dull, pressure, burning, aching, knife-like, "elephant sitting on my chest," ripping, boring, gnawing
- **R**egion/**R**adiation: back, neck, arm, or jaw; substernal, deep, or superficial
- **S**everity: 1 to 10
- **T**iming: constant or intermittent ("Do you have it now?"), pattern with activity

Associated features: dyspnea, nausea, vomiting, diaphoresis, previous history of chest pain, syncope, palpitations, similar to previous MI, change in appetite, history of GERD, abdominal pain, cough, hemoptysis, sputum, dysphagia, cocaine use, rash, neuromuscular weakness, neurologic deficits, recent URI or viral syndrome

Miscellaneous: assessment of risk factors (previous CAD, smoking, DM, family history, HTN), previous visit to cardiologist, history of stress test or catheterization

## Physical Examination

- Fever, hypotension or hypertension, tachycardia or bradycardia, hypoxia, wide pulse pressure, tachypnea, reproducible chest pain, $S_3$, $S_4$, cardiac murmur, JVD, crackles or rhonchi, wheezing, decreased breath sounds, diaphoresis, signs of consolidation, pallor
- Abdominal pain, decreased bowel sounds, rib crepitus, rash, leg erythema, pretibial or sacral edema, hyperpigmentation of the lower extremities, bruising
- CABG scar, saphenous vein scar

## 🔬 Laboratory Studies

■ ECG, CBC, CMP, PT/PTT/INR, UA, UDS, troponin, LDH, myoglobin, CPK/MB, CXR, BNP, D-dimer

■ Consider ABG, chest CT, V/Q, TEE, LE Doppler

## 💊 Management

■ Give ABCs and correct triage

■ Treat underlying disorder

■ Give ASA if there are no contraindications

■ Correct hypovolemia if there are no contraindications

## ✳️ Pearls

■ "Top killer 7": MI, tension pneumothorax, PE, cardiac tamponade, aortic dissection, esophageal rupture, ruptured peptic ulcer

### Differential Diagnosis of Chest Pain: **CHEST PAIN**

**C**ostochondritis/**C**ocaine abuse
**H**erpes zoster/**H**yperventilation
**E**sophagitis/**E**sophageal spasm
**S**tenosis (atrial stenosis)
**T**rauma
**P**E/**P**neumonia/**P**neumothorax/**P**ericarditis/**P**ancreatitis
**A**ngina/**A**ortic dissection/**A**ortic aneurysm
**I**nfarction/**I**ntervertebral disk disease
**N**europsychiatric disorders

---

## Congestive Heart Failure (CHF; Acute Exacerbation)

---

CHF is best summarized as the condition in which cardiac output is unable to meet systemic demands. Patients with acute exacerbations of CHF usually present with acute PE as a result of lung fluid leaking into the pulmonary interstitium from fluid back-up. Systolic CHF can occur from excess afterload or MI. Diastolic CHF results from improper filling of the left ventricle during diastole. Patients with left-sided CHF have dyspnea, orthopnea, PND, fatigue, crackles, and diaphoresis. Patients with right-sided CHF have peripheral edema, JVD, and an hepatojugular reflex.

### Pertinent Positives/Negatives: OPQRST

- **O**nset: length of dyspnea (days, weeks); on heavy exertion, mild exertion, or rest (cause?)
- **P**rovocative/**P**alliative: dyspnea (at rest or on exertion), stress (emotion, exercise, eating), orthopnea (number of pillows), worse at night or when lying flat
- **Q**uality: chest pain (describe)
- **R**egion/**R**adiation: chest pain, dyspnea, leg pain
- **S**everity: 1 to 10
- **T**iming: progressively worse or baseline?

Associated features: history of CHF, MI, or COPD; productive cough; fatigue; palpitations; wheezing; leg swelling; vascular surgery; leg pain; compliance with medication; change in diet ($Na^+$ intake)

#### Causes of CHF: FAILURE

**F**orgot medication
**A**rrhythmia/**A**nemia
**I**schemia/**I**nfarction/**I**nfection
**L**ifestyle: too much salt
**U**pregulation of cardiac output: pregnancy, hyperthyroidism
**R**enal failure
**E**mbolism: pulmonary

## ✍ Physical Examination

■ Fever, hypertension, tachycardia, anxiety, dyspnea, tachypnea, JVD, peripheral edema, sacral edema, CVP, hepatojugular reflex, $S_3$, $S_4$, pulsus alternans, crackles, Cheyne-Stokes respirations

■ RUQ tenderness, cool extremities

## 🔬 Laboratory Studies

■ ECG, CXR, CBC, CMP, cardiac enzymes

■ Consider BNP, digitoxin level, D-dimer, echocardiography

## 💊 Management (Table 3-2)

■ Acute PE
  ■ ABCs
  ■ $O_2$, CPAP, or ETT
  ■ Nitrates, furosemide, morphine
  ■ Consider dopamine or dobutamine

■ CHF
  ■ Vasodilator (NTG or hydralazine)
  ■ ACE inhibitor
  ■ Diuretics
  ■ Consider beta-blocker when acute exacerbation has resolved

## �֎ Pearls

■ Major causes of acute PE: noncompliance, worsening CHF, ischemia

■ CXR findings: pulmonary vasculature enlarged with redistribution to lung apices, Kerley B lines, cardiomegaly

**TABLE 3-2**

## Treatment of CHF and Pulmonary Edema

| Treatment | Mechanism |
|---|---|
| Position: place patient in sitting position with legs dependent | • Increases lung volume and vital capacity<br>• Decreases work of respirations and venous return to the heart |
| Oxygen | • Increases arterial $PO_2$ and causes pulmonary vasodilation<br>• Nonrebreather masks with reservoirs can provide 100% $O_2$<br>• Continuous positive airway pressure (CPAP) can be applied during spontaneous respirations with a tight-fitting mask to help prevent alveolar collapse and improve gas exchange<br>• Intubation if patient cannot maintain adequate oxygenation despite 100% $O_2$ delivery or if signs of cerebral hypoxia (lethargy or obtundation)<br>• Positive end-expiratory pressure (PEEP) can be used to prevent alveolar collapse and improve gas exchange |
| Nitroglycerin | Decreases preload:<br>• Dilates venous capacitance vessels inhibiting venous return to the heart<br>Decreases afterload:<br>• Decreases systemic vascular resistance and facilitates cardiac emptying |

| Loop diuretics (furosemide) | Decrease preload:<br>• Decrease venous tone and increase venous capacitance<br>• Cause diuresis |
|---|---|
| Morphine | Decreases preload:<br>• Dilates the capacitance vessels of peripheral venous bed reducing venous return to central circulation<br>Decreases afterload:<br>• Mild arterial vasodilation |
| Pressors (dopamine, dobutamine) | • Dopamine (pressure too low): If acute pulmonary edema with signs and symptoms of shock and initial SBP <100<br>• Dobutamine (normotensive pump failure): If acute pulmonary edema with SBP >100 |
| Dialysis | • Decreases intravascular volume<br>Useful in renal patients when diuretics are ineffective |
| Digoxin: for patient with CHF and atrial fibrillation | • Slows the conduction through the AV node (controls rate)<br>• Increases both the force and velocity of myocardial contraction (increases pump function) |
| Nitroprusside: for patients with hypertension as cause of pulmonary edema | • Vasodilates both arteriolar and venous beds |

(From Mick N, et al., *Blueprints Emergency Medicine*, 2nd ed. Malden, MA: Blackwell Publishing, 2006.)

## Endocarditis

Endocarditis is an infection of the cardiac valves, the walls of the heart, or the tissue surrounding prosthetic heart valves. Acute endocarditis infects previously normal valves and frequently has more destructive complications (valve incompetence, heart failure). Subacute endocarditis affects abnormal valves. Patients can present with constitutional symptoms or in fulminant heart failure.

### Pertinent Positives/Negatives: OPQRST

- **O**nset: length of symptoms (days, weeks)
- **P**rovocative/**P**alliative: not applicable
- **Q**uality: not applicable
- **R**egion/**R**adiation: not applicable
- **S**everity: 1 to 10
- **T**iming: constancy, previous history of same condition

Associated features: fevers, chills, malaise, fatigue, anorexia, influenza-like syndrome, weight loss, arthralgias, palpitations, dyspnea, chest pain, productive cough, neurologic symptoms (AMS, headache, hemiplegia, blindness), IV drug use, valve replacement, recent dental work, HIV-positive status, dialysis, heart murmur, venous catheters, implantable defibrillator

### Physical Examination

- Fever, tachycardia or bradycardia, hypertension or hypotension, AMS, cardiac murmur (99% present in subacute, 66% in acute; often regurgitant), wide pulse pressure
- Joint tenderness, dermatologic manifestations (20% of cases: Roth spots, splinter hemorrhages, Osler nodes, Janeway

lesions), clubbing, splenomegaly, abdominal pain, IV drug markings

### 🔬 Laboratory Studies

■ ECG, CBC, CMP, blood culture × 2 (consider 3–5), CXR, ESR/CRP, cardiac enzymes

■ Consider echocardiogram (TTE: 60%, TEE: 90% sensitive)

### 💊 Management

■ ABCs

■ Correct hypovolemia (if no contraindications), antibiotics (nafcillin with aminoglycoside, consider vancomycin)

■ Consider surgical care

### 🎯 Pearls

■ *Streptococcus viridans* is the cause in the normal population, *Staphylococcus aureus* in drug users, and *S. epidermidis* in patients with prosthetic valves.

■ The aortic and mitral valves are the most common valves affected, but in IV drug users, right-sided lesions are more common (tricuspid valve).

■ Consider endocarditis in all IV drug users with fever.

■ As many as 50% of positive blood cultures are false positive ("one set is worse than none").

■ Roth spots: retinal hemorrhages

■ Janeway lesions: irregular painless macules on hands and/or feet

■ Osler nodes: small, tender, red or purple nodules on fingers and/or toes

■ Splinter hemorrhages: linear red lines in fingernails

## Hypertension/Hypertensive Emergencies

A hypertensive emergency results from increased BP resulting in end-organ damage or dysfunction. Hypertensive urgency is the elevation of BP to a level that may be harmful (DBP, 115 mm Hg) but without evidence of end-organ damage. Because hypertensive emergencies and urgencies are treated very differently, it is important to exclude hypertensive emergencies quickly and systematically. HTN (nonurgent) can also be classified as primary (essential) or secondary (caused by another condition [i.e., pheochromocytoma, renal artery stenosis]).

### Pertinent Positives/Negatives: OPQRST

- **O**nset: length of history of HTN
- **P**rovocative/**P**alliative: medication compliance
- **Q**uantity: not applicable
- **R**egion/**R**adiation: chest pain, headache, back pain, blurred vision
- **S**everity: 1 to 10
- **T**iming: not applicable

Associated features: history of HTN or heart disease, or kidney disease, dyspnea, diplopia, hemiparesis, seizures, weakness, nausea and/or vomiting, pregnancy (date of LMP), AMS, confusion, cocaine or amphetamine use, thyroid disease, hematuria, oliguria, history of trauma

### 🩺 Physical Examination

- Fever, tachycardia, focal neurologic deficits, AMS, coma or stupor, peripheral pulses, crackles, evidence of CHF, $S_3$ or $S_4$

- JVD, abdominal pulsatile mass
- Funduscopic examination (cotton wool spots, hemorrhage, papilledema)
- BP measurement in both arms

## 🔬 Laboratory Studies

- ECG, CXR, head CT, CBC, CMP (especially BUN/Cr), UA (RBCs, protein), drug screen, cardiac enzymes

## 💊 Management

- ABCs
- Reduce MAP by one third over 30-60 minutes (do not lower below 120 mm Hg) via IV agents (labetalol, NTG, nitroprusside, hydralazine for preeclampsia)
- Consider multiple agents (Table 3-3). The new agent fenoldopam is very useful in renal failure– and cocaine-induced HTN; it works as dopamine antagonist and is cleared in the serum.

## ❋ Pearls

- There are no predetermined criteria for the BP level necessary to induce a hypertensive emergency.
- Mild headache alone with increased BP does not constitute a hypertensive emergency.
- MAP = (2 DBP + SBP)/3
- Avoid beta-blockers in cocaine-induced HTN.
- The most common cause of HTN urgency is noncompliance with medications.

---

### TABLE 3-3

## Agents Used for Hypertensive Emergencies

| Agent | Indications | Contraindications |
|-------|-------------|-------------------|
| Diazoxide | • Malignant hypertension<br>• Hypertensive encephalopathy<br>• Pregnancy-induced hypertension<br>• Preeclampsia or eclampsia | • Aortic dissection<br>• Acute MI |
| Hydralazine | • Eclampsia | |
| Labetalol | • Malignant hypertension<br>• Hypertensive encephalopathy<br>• Aortic dissection | • Beta-blockers |
| Nitroglycerin | • Myocardial ischemia<br>• Congestive heart failure | |
| Nitroprusside | • Malignant hypertension<br>• Hypertensive encephalopathy<br>• Aortic dissection<br>(with beta-blocker) | • Pregnancy |
| Phentolamine | • Agent of choice for excess catecholamine states:<br>  1. Pheochromocytoma<br>  2. MAO inhibitor reactions<br>  3. Cocaine or other stimulants<br>  4. Antihypertensive withdrawal | |

(*From Mick N, et al. Blueprints Emergency Medicine, 2nd ed. Malden, MA: Blackwell Publishing, 2006.*)

---

## Myocardial Infarction (MI)

Ischemic heart disease is the leading cause of death in the United States. Acute MI results from plaque rupture and thrombus formation in a coronary artery, resulting in ischemia, injury, and myocardial necrosis. Classically, patients present with crushing, sudden, substernal chest pain radiating to the jaw, neck, or arm. It is always necessary to be cautious of atypical symptoms (e.g., dyspnea, nausea, diaphoresis, weakness, AMS) in certain patient populations, especially the elderly, women, and people with diabetes. Clinicians should be aware that MI is often *underdiagnosed,* and they should have a strong index of suspicion in any patient who may have cardiac ischemia.

## Pertinent Positives/Negatives: OPQRST

- **O**nset: sudden, subtle, progressive, regressive, insidious, after trauma
- **P**rovocative/**P**alliative: provoking factors (eating, exercise, emotional or physical stress, walking, breathing); palliative factors (NTG and positioning)
- **Q**uality: worsens with exertion, eating, emotion, breathing, stress (emotional or physical), movement of arms or legs; improves with NTG or positioning
- **R**egion/**R**adiation: back, neck, arm, or jaw pain; substernal, deep, or superficial pain
- **S**everity: 1 to 10
- **T**iming: constant or intermittent, ("Do you have it now?"), pattern with activity

Associated features: dyspnea, nausea, vomiting, diaphoresis, previous history of chest pain, syncope, palpitations, similar to previous MI, change in appetite, history of GERD, abdominal pain, cough, hemoptysis, sputum, dysphagia, cocaine use, rash, neuromuscular weakness, neurologic deficits, recent URI or viral syndrome, fever or chills

Miscellaneous: assessment of risk factors (previous CAD, smoking, DM, family history, HTN, hypercholesterolemia), occupation, previous evaluation of chest pain, previous visit to cardiologist, previous stress test or cardiac catheterization

## Physical Examination

- Fever, hypotension or hypertension, tachycardia or brady-cardia, pale appearance, diaphoresis, "angor animi" (feeling of impending doom), cardiac murmur, $S_3$, $S_4$, crackles, JVD, asymmetric expansion of chest, reproducible chest pain, evidence of CHF
- Skin rash, previous CABG or vascular grafting scars

## Laboratory Studies

- ECG, CBC, CMP, PT/PTT/INR, UDS, troponin, LDH, myoglobin, CPK/MB, CXR
- Obtain old records, ECGs, and catheterization reports
- Consider echocardiography

### Causes of ST-Segment Elevation on ECG: ELEVATION

**E**lectrolytes
**L**eft bundle branch block
**E**arly repolarization
**V**entricular hypertrophy
**A**neurysm
**T**reatment (pericardiocentesis)
**I**njury (acute MI, contusion)
**O**sborne waves (hypothermia)
**N**onocclusive vasospasm

### Causes of ST-Segment Depression on ECG: DEPRESSED ST

**D**rooping valve (mitral valve prolapse)
**E**nlargement of LV with strain
**P**otassium loss (hypokalemia)
**R**eciprocal ST depression (in inferior wall acute MI)
**E**mbolism in lungs (PE)
**S**ubendocardial ischemia
**S**ubendocardial infarct

**E**ncephalon hemorrhage (intracranial hemorrhage)
**D**ilated cardiomyopathy
**S**hock
**T**oxicity of digitalis, quinidine

 **Management**

■ ABCs
■ Morphine, oxygen, NTG, ASA (MONA)
■ Beta-blocker, ACE inhibitor, heparin, statins
■ Cardiac catheterization with stenting
■ Consider TPA if cardiac catheterization not available within 2 hours

## Pearls

■ Levine sign: "clutching center of chest with closed fist"
■ As many as 6% of patients with MIs have reproducible chest wall tenderness.
■ Women have atypical chest pain, often only with dyspnea and fatigue.
■ ECG findings (Table 3-4): hyperacute T waves, J-point elevations, ST-segment elevation or depression, T-wave inversion
■ Myoglobin: increases in 1-2 hours, peaks in 4-6 hours, and returns to normal in 24 hours
■ Troponin: increases in 3-6 hours, peaks in 12-24 hours, and returns to normal in 7 days
■ CPK/MB: increases in 4-6 hours, peaks in 12-36 hours, and returns to normal in 3-4 days
■ O BATMAN: **O**xygen, **B**eta-Blockers, **A**SA, **T**hrombolytics, **M**orphine, **A**CE inhibitors, **N**itrates
■ No NTG with Viagra!
■ A normal ECG does not rule out acute MI or ischemia.

## TABLE 3-4

## Localization of Myocardial Infarction

| ECG Changes (ST segments elevations, T-wave inversions, or Q waves) | Area of Infarct | Artery Involved |
|---|---|---|
| II, III, aVF | Inferior | Right coronary artery |
| $V_1$–$V_3$ | Anteroseptal | Left anterior descending |
| $V_2$–$V_4$ | Anterior | Left anterior descending |
| I, aVL, $V_4$, $V_5$, $V_6$ | Lateral | Left circumflex artery |
| $V_1$–$V_2$<br>• Tall R waves with ST segments depressions and tall upright T waves. This usually occurs in association with inferior MI.<br>• Obtain right-sided leads looking for ST segments elevations in $V_4$R. | Posterior | Right posterior descending artery |

(From Mick N, et al. Blueprints Emergency Medicine, 2nd ed. Malden, MA: Blackwell Publishing, 2006.)

## Syncope

Syncope is the sudden transient loss of consciousness that results in the inability to maintain postural tone, usually resolving spontaneously. Near-syncope should be evaluated as syncope. Syncope results from decreased cerebral perfusion from any number of causes, but the most important etiologies to consider are vasovagal, orthostatic, cardiac, and neurologic conditions. The differential diagnosis should include cardiomyopathy, MI, myocardial ischemia, aortic dissection, PE, cardiac arrhythmia, medications, vasovagal syncope, orthostatic hypotension (dehydration, anemia, acute blood loss, vomiting/diarrhea, malnutrition, DM), TIA or CVA, and psychiatric conditions. Other conditions that should be ruled out include carotid sinus hypersensitivity, situational syncope, valvular heart disease, pericardial disease, congenital heart disease, pulmonary hypertension, seizure, subclavian steal syndrome, migraine, and autonomic dysfunction.

## Pertinent Positives/Negatives: OPQRST

It is very important to obtain an extremely detailed history of events preceding syncope (circumstances, positioning, activity, emotions).

- **O**nset: activity before and during syncope, prodrome, sudden, "lights on–lights off"
- **P**rovocative/**P**alliative: ethanol, drug (caffeine, amphetamines, cocaine, heroin), or medication use (antihypertensives, antiarrhythmics); social situations (stressors, lack of sleep); straining, coughing, or defecating at the time of syncope
- **Q**uality: ask whether the patient remembers hitting the ground, the duration of presyncopal symptoms, or the duration of syncope
- **R**egion/**R**adiation: not applicable
- **S**everity: 1 to 10
- **T**iming: previous history of syncope; ask witnesses about convulsions, complaints before syncope, automatisms, ability to focus after waking, and postictal state or confusion

Associated features: syncope, nausea, palpitations, chest pain, dyspnea, back pain, abdominal pain, diaphoresis, headache, neurologic weakness, diplopia, dysarthria, history of cardiac or neurologic disease (especially seizures), family history of syncope or sudden death, single-car MVA, facial or oral trauma, urination or defecation on awakening

### Physical Examination

- Hypotension or hypertension; tachycardia or bradycardia; fever; AMS; evidence of trauma to face, scalp, or extremities (no defensive injuries to hands or knees, lacerations to tongue); palpable abdominal pulsatile mass; orthostatic BP; cardiac murmur; $S_3$; $S_4$; JVD, irregular rhythm; evidence of CHF
- Carotid bruits, motor or sensory deficits, BP measurements in both arms
- Rectal examination: Heme-positive

### Laboratory Studies

- ECG, Accu-Chek, CBC, CMP, drug screen, cardiac enzymes, D-dimer, ethanol level
- Consider CXR, ABG, head CT, carotid Doppler U/S, echocardiography

### Management

- Consider the etiology of syncope.
- If the patient has a high risk of cardiac etiology (age 45 years +, history of ventricular arrhythmias, history of CHF, abnormal ECG), a further evaluation is warranted.
- If the patient is younger and has a benign physical examination and a normal ECG, he or she has a very low risk of morbidity and can be discharged safely with follow-up.

## ❆ Pearls

- Vertigo and dizziness are not considered near-syncope.
- As many as 13% of patients with acute PE develop syncope.
- The history and the physical examination are by far the most important part of the syncope evaluation; a diagnosis can be achieved in up to 80% on the basis of this evidence alone.
- The postictal state is uncommon with syncope, and if present, lasts less than 30 seconds.
- Lacerations on the lateral side of the tongue are almost 100% specific for seizures, not syncope.
- Orthostatic BP measurements:
  - Is there a decrease in SBP of 20 mm Hg or an increase in heart rate of 20 bpm?
  - Is the patient symptomatic during measurement?

San Francisco criteria are high sensitivity and functions better than subjective physician judgment in evaluating patients with syncope for risk stratification and admission: A rule that considers patients with an abnormal ECG, a complaint of shortness of breath, Hct less than 30%, SBP less than 90 mm Hg, or a history of CHF has 96% (95% confidence interval [CI] 92% to 100%) sensitivity and 62% (95% CI 58% to 66%) specificity. If applied to this cohort, the rule has the potential to decrease the admission rate by 10%.

## Vascular Diseases (AAAs, TAAs)

An aneurysm can be classified as an atherosclerotic aneurysm or a dissecting aneurysm. An arteriosclerotic artery has a thinned tunica media with decreased elastin fibers, leading to formation of an aneurysm. A dissecting aneurysm occurs when a tear forms in the intima of the aorta, allowing the blood to "dissect" the layers of the arterial wall, creating a true and false lumen. Dissecting aneurysms are usually the result of hypertension. Patients may present in many ways; they may be unresponsive or in pain, or the aneurysms may be found incidentally. Aneurysms may be thoracic or abdominal.

## Pertinent Positives/Negatives: OPQRST

- **O**nset: sudden onset, abrupt, gradual, after trauma, drug use
- **P**rovocative/**P**alliative: worse with positioning
- **Q**uality: ripping, sharp, or tearing pain
- **R**egion/**R**adiation: chest, back, abdominal, flank, neck or arm, or leg pain
- **S**everity: 1 to 10
- **T**iming: constant or intermittent

Associated features: pulsatile mass, nausea or vomiting, syncope, family history of aneurysms, peripheral vascular disease, Marfan syndrome, smoking, neuromuscular weakness, cocaine use, bicuspid aortic valve, history of Ehlers-Danlos syndrome, trauma, third trimester of pregnancy or postpartum

## Physical Examination

- Hypotension or hypertension, tachycardia, pulsatile abdominal mass, wide pulse pressure, pulsus paradoxus, peripheral pulses, focal neurologic deficits (thoracic), hemiplegia, BP discrepancies in both arms and legs, cardiac murmur

## Laboratory Studies

- CXR, AAS, ECG, CBC, CMP, PT/PTT/INR, UA, type and cross for PRBCs
- Consider abdominal U/S (unstable) vs. CT (stable) vs. echocardiogram vs. MRI vs. aortography

## Management

- ABCs
- Correct hypovolemia

■ Abdominal

　■ Take to OR

■ Thoracic

　■ Control hypotension (SBP ~90 mm Hg)

　■ Take to OR if unstable

## 🎯 Pearls

■ CXR findings of thoracic aneurysm include widened mediastinum, obliteration of aortic knob, tracheal deviation, obliteration of aortopulmonary window, deviation of esophagus to right (best seen with NG tube), widened paratracheal stripe, apical cap, left hemothorax, and depressed left mainstream bronchus.

■ *Always* suspect AAA in an older patient with new-onset flank pain and hematuria.

■ Order CT, not IVP, for renal colic.

■ On autopsy, death from AAA is most often misdiagnosed as renal colic.

## 📖 Literature

■ Albers GW, Dalen JE, Laupacis A, et al. Antithrombotic therapy in atrial fibrillation. *Chest*. 2001 Jan;119(1 Suppl): 194S–206S. The authors reviewed the current literature and concluded that the annual stroke risk in AF was 4.5% for patients in a control group and 1.4% for patients taking warfarin.

■ Carpenter CR. Evidence-based emergency medicine/ rational clinical examination abstract. Abdominal palpation for the diagnosis of abdominal aortic aneurysm. *Ann Emerg Med*. 2005;45(5):556–558.

■ Davey MJ. A randomized controlled trial of magnesium sulfate, in addition to usual care, for rate control in atrial fibrillation. *Ann Emerg Med.* 2005;45(4):347–353. This article reported that addition of IV magnesium and digoxin to traditional therapy almost doubles the reduction in recurrent rapid ventricular response.

■ Elpidoforos S, Soteriades JC, Evans, Larson MG, et al. Incidence and Prognosis of Syncope. *N Engl J Med.* 2002; 347(12):878–885. The authors reported that patients diagnosed with vasovagal syncope have a benign prognosis, whereas those with cardiac syncope are at increased risk of death from any causes as well as cardiac death.

■ Hagan PG, Nienaber CA, Isselbacher EM, et al. *JAMA.* 2000 Feb 16;283(7):897–903. The International Registry of Acute Aortic Dissection (IRAD): new insights into an old disease. This article summarized sudden onset of severe sharp pain was the most common presenting complaint, but the clinical presentation was diverse (normal CXR and ECG in 12.4% and 31.3% of patients, respectively).

■ McSweeney JC, Cody M, O'Sullivan P, et al. Women's Early Warning Signs of Acute Myocardial Infarction *Circulation* (2003). (http://circ.ahajournals.org/cgi/content/abstract•/108/21/2619). This article identified that almost 50% of women diagnosed with acute MI never described classic chest pain.

■ Knudsen CW, Omland T, Clopton P, et al. Diagnostic and prognostic usefulness of natriuretic peptides in emergency department patients with dyspnea. *Am J Med.* 2004; 116(6):363–368. BNP more accurately predicts CHF than history, physical examination, or CXR.

■ Maisel AS, Krishnaswamy P, Nowak RM, et al., for the Breathing Not Properly Multinational Study Investigators. Rapid Measurement of B-Type Natriuretic Peptide in the Emergency Diagnosis of Heart Failure. *N Engl J Med.* 2002;347(14):1126. This article showed that measurement of BNP is useful in establishing or excluding the diagnosis of CHF in patients with acute dyspnea and is more sensitive than physical examination. BNP is elevated first, then changes on CXR are seen, then crackles and/or peripheral edema are found.

■ Milner KA, Vaccarino V, Arnold AL, et al. Gender and age differences in chief complaints of acute myocardial infarction (Worcester Heart Attack Study). *Am J Cardiol.* 2004;93(5):606–608. In this study, the authors reported that the second most common chief complaint (after chest pain) is respiratory symptoms; almost one-fourth of women and men had this chief complaint. Younger women were two times more likely to present with respiratory symptoms as their chief complaint compared with men in the same age group. A large proportion of patients, including almost half of the women, who were ultimately diagnosed with acute MI, did not present with a chief complaint of chest pain. The presence of comorbid conditions decreases the likelihood of having chest pain as a chief complaint and explains most of the gender differences in presentation, particularly in younger patients.

■ Norman PE, Jamrozik K, Lawrence-Brown MM, et al. *BMJ.* 2004;329(7477):1259. Population-based randomized controlled trial on impact of screening on mortality from abdominal aortic aneurysm. These articles showed that screening examinations do lower AAA mortality and that physical examination is a poor means of detecting the aneurysm. On physical examination, less than half of all high-risk patients suspected of having an enlarged aorta are found to have an AAA, and only one fourth of those are at high risk for rupture (>5 cm). Therefore, when a ruptured abdominal aortic aneurysm is suspected, imaging studies should be performed regardless of physical examination findings. Both obesity and abdominal examination not specifically directed at measuring aortic width appear to reduce the sensitivity of abdominal palpation in detecting AAAs.

- Quinn JV. The San Francisco Syncope Rule vs physician judgment and decision making. *Am J Emerg Med.* 2005 Oct 1;23(6):782–786. Derivation of the San Francisco Syncope Rule to predict patients with short-term serious outcomes. *Ann Emerg Med.* 2004;43(2):224–232.

- Shapiro SM, Young E, De Guzman S, et al. Transesophageal echocardiography in diagnosis of infective endocarditis. *Chest.* 1994 Feb;105(2):377–382. This article reported that TEE was significantly more sensitive than TTE and highly specific in both confirming the clinical diagnosis of infective endocarditis as well as in identifying valvular vegetations in patients at risk of this infection.

- Sohail MR. Medical versus surgical management of *Staphylococcus aureus* prosthetic valve endocarditis. *Am J Med.* 2006 Feb 1;119(2):147–154. Patients with *S. aureus* endocarditis and prosthetic valves need surgery; mortality was 50% for those patients who received medical therapy compared with 28% for those who received surgical treatment.

- Stone GW, Grimes CL, O'Neil WW. Primary coronary angioplasty versus thrombolysis. *N Engl J Med.* 1997 Oct 16;337(16):1168–1170. The GUSTO IIB trial showed that primary PTCA was more effective than thrombolytic therapy in reducing death, reinfarction, and stroke, with the greatest benefit in patients who were highest risk.

- U.S. Department of Health and Human Services, National Institutes of Health. Seventh Report of the Joint National Committee on Prevention, Detection, Evaluation, and Treatment of High Blood Pressure (JNC 7) Boston, MA. (2003). These guidelines recommended that thiazide-type diuretics, either alone or combined with drugs from other classes, be used in drug treatment for most patients with uncomplicated hypertension. Certain high-risk conditions are compelling indications for the initial use of other antihypertensive drug classes. The JNC 7 also stated that most patients with hypertension require at least two agents to achieve goal BP.

# 4 Gastrointestinal System

## Abdominal Pain

Evaluating a patient with abdominal pain can be quite challenging because of the many causes. The differential diagnosis includes the following conditions, which should always be excluded: aortic aneurysm, MI, ectopic pregnancy, obstruction, mesenteric ischemia, appendicitis, perforated peptic ulcer, splenic rupture, testicular torsion, ovarian torsion, and PID (Table 4-1). Be aware of a shift in differential diagnosis based on the patient's age and sex.

### Pertinent Positives/Negatives: OPQRST

- **O**nset: sudden, slow, or insidious; could be postprandial (length of time after meals?)
- **P**rovocative/**P**alliative: improves with food or drink, movement, coughing, postdefecation, medications (antacids)
- **Q**uality: gassy, crampy, sharp, vague, boring (to back), burning, colicky pain; previous history of same abdominal pain
- **R**egion/**R**adiation: location of pain, ask whether pain migrates or radiates
- **S**everity: 1 to 10; duration: intermittent, minutes versus hours, awakens patient at night
- **T**iming: constant or intermittent

Associated features: fever or chills, nausea and/or vomiting, diarrhea or constipation, loose bowel movements, dysuria or

**TABLE 4-1**

## Differential Diagnosis of Abdominal Pain

Common: chronic nonspecific abdominal pain, psychogenic, constipation, dysmenorrhea, mittelschmerz

Less Common: PUD, inflammatory bowel disease, UTI, hernias, medication side effect

Uncommon: appendicitis, biliary tract disease, SBO, salpingitis, ovarian cysts, ectopic pregnancy, miscarriage, pancreatitis, diverticular disease, endometriosis, abdominal angina/mesenteric ischemia

Pancreatitis: gallstones, alcohol abuse, medications (thiazides, antibiotics, antiepileptics, estrogens, steroids, NSAIDs, amiodarone), hypercalcemia, hypertriglyceridemia, post-ERCP, trauma, viral, idiopathic

frequency, scrotal pain, bloating, rectal or vaginal bleeding, anorexia or appetite versus normal appetite

Miscellaneous: LMP, previous surgeries (especially abdominal), alcohol use, history of GERD, trauma, shoulder or groin pain, presence of hernia, history of DM (last Accu-Chek), recent instrumentation, cardiac history (especially AF)

### Differential Diagnosis of Abdominal Pain: ABDOMENAL PANE (abdominal pain)

**A**cute rheumatic fever
**B**lood (purpura, hemolytic crisis)
**D**KA
**CO**llagen vascular disease
**M**igraine (abdominal migraine)
**E**pilepsy (abdominal epilepsy)
**N**ephron (uremia)
**A**bdominal angina
**L**ead

**P**orphyria
**A**rsenic
**N**SAIDs
**E**nteric fever

## Physical Examination
- General: patient movement (sitting still or writhing)
- Fever, hypertension or hypotension, tachycardia or brady-cardia
- Distension, surgical scars, high-pitched sounds, diminished bowel sounds, area of maximal tenderness (with and without distraction), palpable mass, peritoneal irritation (muscle guarding/rebound tenderness), CVA tenderness, crackles and/or rhonchi, scleral icterus
- Rectal/pelvic examination: stool guaiac

## Laboratory Studies
- CBC, CMP, amylase/lipase, UA, UDS, β-hCG, CXR/AAS, wet prep, GC/chlamydia
- Consider ECG, ESR, CRP, CT, U/S

## Management
- Treat underlying condition
- Correct hypovolemia

## Pearls
- In every woman with abdominal pain, rule out ectopic pregnancy (β-hCG).
- Elderly patients with abdominal pain are much more likely to have serious pathology.

■ Ask patients if they are hungry (offer food, meal) to evaluate for anorexia.

■ Be aware that acute angle glaucoma can present as abdominal pain with nausea and/or vomiting as its only symptom.

■ Use of chronic steroids may hide serious abdominal pathology.

■ Top life-threatening causes of abdominal pain: aneurysm, appendicitis, ectopic pregnancy, mesenteric ischemia, small bowel obstruction, perforation, intussusception, peritonitis

## Appendicitis

Appendicitis is inflammation of the vermiform appendix that can progress to perforation. This disorder has varying presentations and can mimic other disease processes, and no single sign, symptom, or laboratory test can make the diagnosis of appendicitis in all cases. Patients can present at any time during the disease process, and morbidity increases with diagnostic delay. Classically, patients present with dull periumbilical pain that waxes and wanes followed by nausea and/or vomiting and anorexia. The pain then shifts to the RLQ and becomes sharp, progressively worse, and continuous until perforation, which presents as an acute abdomen and/or peritonitis.

### Pertinent Positives/Negatives: OPQRST

■ **O**nset: sudden or subtle onset of pain

■ **P**rovocative/**P**alliative: improves with positioning (guarding), food or drink, "horrible bumpy ride," possible pain resolution after emesis

■ **Q**uality: vague periumbilical pain, sharp RLQ pain

■ **R**egion/**R**adiation: may be RLQ or periumbilical; may migrate or radiate, associated with fever, nausea and vomiting (pain before or after vomiting), loose stools, constipation, anorexia, dysuria, frequency, flank or back pain, vaginal bleeding or discharge, rectal bleeding, testicular pain, penile discharge, hematuria

■ **S**everity: 1 to 10

■ **T**iming: constant or intermittent

Miscellaneous: first day of LMP, cardiac history (AF), last meal, similar symptoms with family members, surgical history, "bulge" or hernia

### RLQ Pain: APPENDICITIS

**A**ppendicitis/**A**bscess
**P**ID/**P**eriod
**P**ancreatitis
**E**ctopic/**E**ndometriosis
**N**eoplasia
**D**iverticulitis
**I**ntussusception
**C**rohn disease/**C**yst (ovarian)
**I**nflammatory bowel disease
**T**orsion (ovary)
**I**rritable bowel syndrome
**S**tones

 **Physical Examination**

■ General: lying still in comfort or writhing in pain

■ Fever, tachycardia, hypertension or hypotension, guarding (involuntary vs. voluntary), RLQ tenderness, rigidity, pain on percussion, rebound tenderness, pain with cough, abdominal distension, hyperactive or hypoactive bowel

sounds, hernias, abdominal surgical scars, CVA tenderness, Murphy sign, McBurney point tenderness, crackles or rhonchi
▪ Rectal examination, testicular examination, pelvic examination with adnexal fullness/tenderness
▪ Peritoneal irritation: rebound tenderness, percussion of patient's heel, hit the bed hard to elicit pain
▪ Rovsing sign: RLQ pain with palpation of LLQ
▪ Psoas sign: RLQ pain with hyperextension of right hip
▪ Obturator sign: RLQ pain with internal rotation of flexed right hip

## Laboratory Studies
▪ CBC, CMP, β-hCG, UA, AAS
▪ Consider CRP, CT, U/S, barium enema (Fig. 4-1)

## Management
▪ Correct hypovolemia
▪ NPO, analgesia, IV antibiotics
▪ Surgical evaluation

## Pearls
▪ Administering analgesics is safe in abdominal pain and does not adversely effect diagnostic evaluation.
▪ Vomiting that precedes pain suggests intestinal obstruction, not appendicitis.
▪ Be aware that an inflamed appendix can cause irritation to local tissues (pancreas, ureters, bowel), resulting in dysfunction (positive UA, increased amylase/lipase, localized ileus).

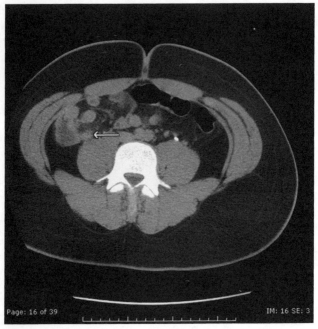

**Figure 4-1** Typical CT findings in appendicitis. A very small "target" sign is visible near the arrow, with surrounding fat stranding. (*Courtesy of Children's Hospital Boston, Boston, Massachusetts.*)

- A CBC is nonspecific and can miss as many as 4% of cases.
- Appendicitis in late pregnancy can present with RUQ pain.
- Incidence peaks in people 10–30 years of age.

## Cirrhosis/End-Stage Liver Disease/Encephalopathy

Cirrhosis is a generic term for an end-stage of chronic liver disease. It is characterized by the destruction of hepatocytes, with replacement of fibrotic tissue. There are multiple causes of cirrhosis, with infectious, drug induced, and alcohol-induced being the most common. Hepatic encephalopathy is a manifestation of cirrhosis, with complex pathophysiology that results in disordered cerebral function. Cirrhosis has multiple sequelae, including bleeding diathesis, ascites, spontaneous bacterial peritonitis, hepatorenal syndrome, and esophageal varices.

## Pertinent Positives/Negatives: OPQRST

■ **O**nset: sudden or subtle onset of symptoms; similar to previous episodes of encephalopathy/worsening ascites

■ **P**rovocative/**P**alliative: worsens with abdominal pain, fever or chills, being out of medications; improves with medication compliance

■ **Q**uality: possible pain

■ **R**egion/**R**adiation: associated with AMS or confusion, abdominal pain, nausea and/or vomiting, melena, hematochezia, or hematemesis, increased abdominal girth, easy bruising or bleeding, gynecomastia, jaundice, edema, color changes in urine or stool

■ **S**everity: 1 to 10

■ **T**iming: constant or intermittent

Miscellaneous: previous history of liver disease (see Hepatitis), medications (acetaminophen), IV drug use, ascites (new vs. old), alcohol use

### Causes of Cirrhosis: HEPATIC

**H**emochromatosis (primary)
**E**nzyme deficiency (alpha-1-antitrypsin)
**P**osthepatic (infection + drug induced)
**A**lcoholic
**T**yrosinosis
**I**ndian childhood (galactosemia)
**C**ardiac/**C**holestatic (biliary)/**C**ancer/**C**opper (Wilson disease)

### Physical Examination

- Fever, tachycardia or bradycardia, hypotension
- Evidence of liver disease (spider angioma, palmar erythema, gynecomastia, testicular atrophy, ascites), jaundice, AMS, asterixis, fetor hepaticus, superficial bruising, ascites, muscle wasting, abdominal pain, edema
- Rectal examination (positive guaiac)

### Laboratory Studies

- CBC, CMP with liver enzymes, ammonia, PT/PTT/INR, UA
- Consider ammonia level, ascitic fluid analysis

### Management

- Correct fluid or electrolyte abnormality, paracentesis, low-sodium diet with diuretic, beta-blocker, vitamin K supplementation, treat sequelae
- Consider lactulose if occurs with encephalopathy

### Pearls

- Some say serum ammonia levels do not correlate with hepatic encephalopathy (see Literature).
- Do not remove large quantities of ascitic fluid, because it may result in electrolyte abnormalities.

## Gallbladder Disease

Gallbladder disease includes many different clinical entities, including cholelithiasis, cholecystitis, and cholangitis. Cholelithiasis (and the resulting biliary colic) are caused by the transient cystic duct blockage from impacted stones. Classically, they present with postprandial RUQ pain, radiating to the shoulder or scapula. Cholecystitis is the obstruction of the cystic duct, resulting in distention, inflammation, and possibly infection. Cholangitis is the infection of the biliary tree and is a surgical emergency.

## Pertinent Positives/Negatives: OPQRST

- **O**nset: sudden or subtle onset of symptoms; similar to previous "gallbladder pain"
- **P**rovocative/**P**alliative: postprandial pain, self-limiting, worse with fatty foods
- **Q**uantity: sharp, stabbing, or colicky RUQ pain
- **R**egion/**R**adiation: radiates to the shoulder or scapula
- **S**everity: 1 to 10
- **T**iming: constant or intermittent pain

Associated features: fevers or chills, nausea or vomiting, hematemesis, flatulence, anorexia, jaundice, pruritus, confusion or AMS, dizziness

Miscellaneous: family history of gallbladder disease, alcohol or drug use, history of heart disease, pregnancy

### Differential Diagnosis of Acute Cholangitis: CHOLANGITIS

**C**harcot triad/**C**onjugated bilirubin increase
**H**epatic abscesses/**H**epatic (intra/extra) bile ducts/**H**LA B8, DR3
**O**bstruction
**L**eukocytosis
**A**lkaline phosphatase increase
**N**eoplasms
**G**allstones
**I**nflammatory bowel disease (ulcerative colitis)
**T**ransaminase increase
**I**nfection
**S**clerosing

## Physical Examination

- Fever, hypotension, tachycardia
- Obvious pain vs. comfort, abdominal discomfort, peritoneal signs, Murphy sign (tenderness and inspiratory pause elicited during palpation of RUQ during deep breath), distended or palpable gallbladder, AMS, flank pain, surgical scars

## Laboratory Studies

- CBC, CMP with LFTs, UA
- Consider ECG, cardiac enzymes, amylase/lipase, PT/PTT/INR, blood cultures, U/S, HIDA scan, CT

## Management

- Acute cholecystitis: IV antibiotics (ampicillin, sulbactam), fluid replacement, NG tube, analgesia, surgical intervention
- Acute cholangitis: IV antibiotics (ampicillin, aminoglycoside, clindamycin); fluid replacement; THC, ERCP, or surgery

## Pearls

- Twenty percent of gallstones are radiopaque.
- Gas in the biliary tree is evidence supporting the presence of cholangitis.
- Charcot triad of acute cholangitis: RUQ, fever, jaundice
- Reynolds pentad: Charcot triad (RUQ, fever, jaundice), hypotension, AMS

### 5 Fs of Gallbladder Disease

**F**emale

**F**at

**F**orty

**F**ertile

**F**latulent

## Hepatitis

Hepatitis is the inflammation of the liver secondary to a number of causes, but the majority of cases result from either a viral etiology or are induced by alcohol. It is also necessary to rule out toxins (especially acetaminophen), parasites, and autoimmune causes. Presentations vary, depending on etiology, but patients commonly have RUQ tenderness, weakness, anorexia, nausea and/or vomiting, and possibly jaundice.

### Pertinent Positives/Negatives: OPQRST

■ **O**nset: subtle or sudden onset of symptoms; previous history of liver disease or hepatitis

■ **P**rovocative/**P**alliative: worsens with alcohol

■ **Q**uality: not applicable

■ **R**egion/**R**adiation: not applicable

■ **S**everity: 1 to 10

■ **T**iming: constant or intermittent

Associated features: abdominal pain, malaise, arthralgia, URI symptoms, nausea and vomiting, fatigue, jaundice, change in bowel patterns or color, change in color of urine, anorexia, increased abdominal girth, AMS or confusion

Miscellaneous: history of contact with hepatitis, blood transfusions, immunization status, occupation, IV drug use, tattoos, sexual history, pregnant, recent travel, sanitation, alcohol use, medication use (isoniazid, acetaminophen)

## Physical Examination
■ Fever, tachycardia, hypertension or hypotension
■ Jaundice, evidence of cirrhosis (palmar erythema, spider angiomas, testicular atrophy, gynecomastia), RUQ tenderness, hepatosplenomegaly, dark urine, edema, scleral icterus, evidence of IV drug use

## Laboratory Studies
■ Hepatitis serologies, CBC, CMP, liver enzymes (ALT > AST), PT/PTT/INR, UA, ammonia

## Management
■ Supportive care, correct electrolyte abnormalities
■ Consider interferon or steroids

## Pearls
■ Hepatitis C is the most common cause of viral hepatitis in the US (more contagious than HIV).
■ Jaundice appears to the naked eye at serum bilirubin of 3 mg/dL.
■ In dark-skinned individuals, check under the tongue for jaundice.

## Hernia

A hernia is simply the protrusion of a structure through a wall defect. There are many types of abdominal wall hernias, including inguinal, femoral, umbilical, incisional, and spigelian. Besides the type, the hernias should be classified as either **reducible** (contents can be pushed back to original position), **incarcerated** (not able to be reduced, can be acute or chronic), or **strangulated** (incarcerated with vascular compromise). Patients usually present with a history of a "bulge" or lump or may be septic from an incarcerated hernia.

## Pertinent Positives/Negatives: OPQRST

■ **O**nset: sudden or subtle pain, previous episodes of similar pain or "bulge"

■ **P**rovocative/**P**alliative: worsens with coughing, sit-ups, flexing trunk, Valsalva maneuver; improves with positioning, ability to push the "bulge" back

■ **Q**uality: description of pain

■ **R**egion/**R**adiation: radiating pain

■ **S**everity: 1 to 10

■ **T**iming: constant or intermittent

Associated features: fever and chills, nausea and vomiting, increased abdominal girth, appetite or anorexia, melena or hematochezia, back pain, urinary symptoms

Miscellaneous: location of hernia, previous abdominal surgeries (including hernia repair), pregnancy, DM, occupation (heavy lifting)

 Physical Examination

■ Fever, hypotension, tachycardia

■ Abdominal pain, reducible or nonreducible hernia, bowel sounds (hyper/hypoactive), previous surgical scars, peritoneal signs

■ Rectal examination: possible blood or a mass

**Laboratory Studies**

- CBC, CMP, AAS, UA, β-hCG, LDH
- Consider CT

**Management**

- Correct hypovolemia, treat SBO if present.
- Reduce if possible. If the hernia is reducible, avoid heavy lifting or straining. Consider surgical intervention. *Do not attempt to reduce dead bowel into the abdomen.*

**Pearls**

- Bowel obstruction can be the first presenting sign of a hernia.
- Direct inguinal hernia: protrudes through floor of Hesselbach's triangle; from weakness in abdominal musculature
- Indirect inguinal hernia: most common in all sexes and ages; lateral to inferior epigastric artery; hernia sac can travel into scrotum; from patent processus vaginalis (congenital)
- Femoral hernia: common in women, hernia protrudes through femoral ring; most susceptible to incarceration
- Incisional hernia: common after any wound (usually surgical)

## Jaundice

Jaundice is the yellowish discoloration of the skin and/or mucous membranes caused by elevated levels of serum bilirubin. It may be a presenting complaint from the patient

### TABLE 4-2

## Differential Diagnosis of Jaundice

Neonatal: ABO incompatibility, sepsis, hepatic (Gilbert disease, Crigler-Najjar syndrome), TORCH (toxoplasmosis, rubella, cytomegalovirus, herpes simplex, syphilis), anatomic defect, toxins, breast-milk, hypothyroidism, physiologic

Adult: hepatitis (viral, autoimmune, drug-induced), obstructive (infection, tumor, gallstones), cirrhosis, pancreatic carcinoma, primary biliary cirrhosis, acute cholangitis, hemolysis, transfusion reaction, Wilson disease, hemochromatosis, cholestasis, primary sclerosis cholangitis, pancreatitis

or an abnormal finding on physical examination. Jaundice is easier to detect in lighter pigmented individuals. Patients with a darker complexion often have hyperpigmented sclera, and this can be confused with scleral icterus. Jaundice is the presentation of many conditions, and it is important to exclude life-threatening causes immediately (Table 4-2).

### Pertinent Positives/Negatives: OPQRST

■ **O**nset: sudden or subtle onset of jaundice; possible history of jaundice

■ **P**rovocative/**P**alliative: worsens with abdominal pain, anorexia, nausea and/or vomiting, medications

■ **Q**uality: possible pain

■ **R**egion/**R**adiation: not applicable

■ **S**everity: 1 to 10

■ **T**iming: constant or intermittent

Associated features: fevers or chills, recent infection or illness, changes in stool color, ascites, anorexia or appetite changes, fatigue, night sweats, weight loss, pruritus, confusion or AMS, back pain

Miscellaneous: family history of jaundice, sickle cell disease, stool color changes, recent drug ingestion (acetaminophen, isoniazid, ASA), IV drug use, tobacco and alcohol use, blood transfusions, hematologic disorders, history of autoimmune disease, heart failure, congenital errors of metabolism, mushroom ingestion, sexual history, HIV-positive status, history of gallbladder disease, pancreatitis, pregnancy

## Physical Examination

■ Fever, tachycardia, bradycardia, hypotension

■ AMS, cachexia, jaundice, scleral icterus, mucous membrane discoloration (look under tongue), evidence of end-stage liver disease (spider angioma, palmar erythema, ascites, gynecomastia), Murphy's sign, evidence of IV drug use, abdominal pain, surgical scars, fetor hepaticus, alcohol on breath, abdominal mass, JVD, pedal edema, varices, Charcot triad, Reynolds pentad

## Laboratory Studies

■ CBC, CMP with liver enzymes, AAS, UA, PT/PTT/INR, UDS, β-hCG, blood alcohol level, amylase, lipase, acetaminophen

■ Consider GGT, fractionated alkaline phosphatase, RUQ U/S, abdominal CT, HIDA scan

 ## Management

■ Treat underlying cause

## ❄ Pearls

■ Painless jaundice is pancreatic cancer until proven otherwise.

■ Scleral icterus can appear at a serum bilirubin of 2 mg/dL.

## Pancreatitis

Pancreatitis results from inflammation and autodigestion of the gland by pancreatic enzymes. Chronic pancreatitis is the result of recurrent attacks, causing irreversible parenchymal damage and leading to dysfunction. Acute pancreatitis has several causes; the leading ones are alcohol, gallstones, trauma, hypercalcemia, hypertriglyceridemia, viral infections, ERCP, and drugs (especially thiazide diuretics). Patients typically present with sudden-onset, deep, "boring," epigastric pain, radiating to the back, with nausea and vomiting. Pancreatitis can be potentially fatal, with serious sequelae (ARDS, shock).

### Pertinent Positives/Negatives: OPQRST

■ **O**nset: sudden or subtle onset; similar to previous episodes of abdominal pain or pancreatitis

■ **P**rovocative/**P**alliative: worsens with eating, drinking, or alcohol use; improves with positioning and postemesis

■ **Q**uality: burning, boring pain

■ **R**egion/**R**adiation: radiates to back, flank, abdominal quadrants; associated with fevers, night sweats, weight loss, nausea and/or vomiting, urinary symptoms, back pain, anorexia, hematemesis, hematochezia or melena

■ **S**everity: 1 to 10

■ **T**iming: constant or intermittent

Miscellaneous: alcohol use, gallbladder disease, postprandial pain, history of hyperlipidemia and/or hypercholesterolemia, medications (antibiotics, diuretics, steroids, NSAIDs), history of AF, history of cancer, ascites, history of peptic ulcer disease, AMS, history of DM

---

### Differential Diagnosis of Pancreatitis: I GET SMASHED

**I**diopathic
**G**allstones
**E**thanol
**T**rauma
**S**teroids
**M**umps
**A**utoimmune
**S**corpion stings
**H**yperlipidemia/ **H**ypercalcemia
**E**RCP
**D**rugs (including azathioprine and diuretics)

## Physical Examination

- Fever, hypotension, bradycardia or tachycardia
- AMS, smell of alcohol, vomiting, abdominal pain, peritoneal signs, CVA tenderness, jaundice, hyper- or hypoactive bowel sounds, crackles or rhonchi, decreased breath sounds, abdominal bloating, dyspnea, diminished breath sounds
- Grey Turner sign: bluish discoloration of the flanks
- Cullen sign: bluish discoloration of umbilical area

## Laboratory Studies

- CBC, amylase, lipase, CMP, LFTs, LDH, AAS (perforation, sentinel loop, diffuse calcifications), U/S
- Consider CT

**Ranson Criteria for Pancreatitis (at admission): GA LAW**

**G**lucose > 200 mg/dL
**A**ST > 250 U/L
**L**DH > 350 U/L
**A**ge > 55 years
**W**BC > 16,000 mm$^3$

**Ranson Criteria for Pancreatitis (after 48 hours): C & HOBBS (Calvin and Hobbes)**

**C**alcium < 8 mg/dL
**H**ct decrease > 10%
**O**xygen < 60 mm
**B**UN increase > 5 mg/dL
**B**ase deficit > 4 mEq/L
**S**equestration of fluid > 6 L

### Management (Fig. 4-2)

■ ABCs, correct hypovolemia, NPO status (bowel rest), NG tube, analgesia
■ Consider antibiotics, surgical intervention
■ Evaluate for Ranson criteria

### Pearls

■ Grey-Turner sign (blue-black flanks) and Cullen sign (blue-black umbilicus) are evidence of retroperitoneal hemorrhage and severe pancreatitis.
■ Ranson criteria (mortality rates correlate with number of criteria present)
■ A sentinel loop is distention and/or air fluid levels near a site of abdominal pathology.

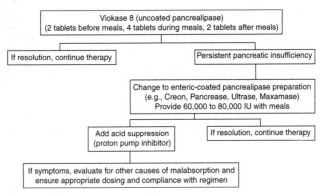

**Figure 4-2** Suggested algorithm for management of pancreatic insufficiency. (*From Lin T and Rypkema S. The Washington Manual of Ambulatory Therapeutics. Philadelphia: Lippincott Williams & Wilkins: 2002:322.*)

- Lipase is much more specific for pancreatic tissue pathology than amylase.
- Watch for complications of pseudocyst (drain surgically if symptomatic) and pancreatic abscess (antibiotics and surgical drainage) several weeks after initial presentation.

## Peptic Ulcer Disease

Peptic ulcer disease is a result of damage to gastric or duodenal mucosa. It can be caused by decreased mucosal defense (medication), bacterial infection (*Helicobacter pylori*), stress (trauma or burns), or increased acid. Patients can present within a spectrum, from a chronic burning abdominal pain to severe sudden abdominal pain (perforated ulcer). The disease is often relieved by antacids or milk.

## Pertinent Positives/Negatives: OPQRST

■ **O**nset: sudden or subtle onset of pain, temporal relationship to food (immediately after food intake or several hours later), change in pain from previous episodes

■ **P**rovocative/**P**alliative: worse or better with food, drink, alcohol, spicy foods

■ **Q**uality: obtain description of pain

■ **R**egion/**R**adiation: radiates to back or abdominal quadrant, associated with melena or hematochezia, nausea and/or vomiting, anorexia

■ **S**everity: 1 to 10

■ **T**iming: constant or intermittent

Miscellaneous: fever, history of GERD, previous surgical history, ASA or NSAID use, alcohol or tobacco use, history of liver disease, pregnant

### Physical Examination

■ Fever, hypertension or hypotension, bradycardia or tachycardia

■ Abdominal pain or tenderness, radiation, peritoneal signs, abdominal surgical scars, CVA tenderness

■ Rectal examination: Heme positive

### Laboratory Studies

■ AAS, CBC, BMP, amylase, lipase, testing for *H. pylori*

■ Consider endoscopy

### Management

■ ABCs, correct hypovolemia, consider NG tube, antibiotics

■ Avoid substances that aggravate pain

**TABLE 4-3**

**Recommended Protocols for Eradication of *Helicobacter pylori***

| |
|---|
| Triple therapies (14-day therapy recommended) |
| Omeprazole, 20 mg PO bid; lansoprazole, 30 mg PO bid; rabeprazole, 20 mg PO bid; or ranitidine bismuth citrate, PO bid |
| *and* two of the following: |
| Amoxicillin, 1 g PO bid |
| Clarithromycin, 500 mg PO bid |
| Metronidazole, 500 mg PO bid |
| Quadruple therapy (7–14 day therapy recommended—longer duration of therapy may have slight cure rate advantage) |
| Omeprazole, 20 mg PO bid; lansoprazole, 30 mg PO bid; or rabeprazole, 30 mg PO bid |
| Tetracycline, 500 mg PO qid |
| Metronidazole, 500 mg PO tid |
| Bismuth subsalicylate, 2 tablets PO qid |

(*Adapted from DY Graham. Therapy of* Helicobacter pylori: *current status and issues.* Gastroenterology *2000;118:S2–S8.*)

- Give antacids, $H_2$ receptor blockers, PPIs, eradication of *H. pylori* (Table 4-3)
- If peritoneal signs, surgical management

## Pearls

- Gastric ulcer pain: shortly after eating
- Duodenal ulcer pain: 2–3 hours after eating
- Obstruction can occur after an ulcer heals.

■ Biopsy all gastric ulcers to exclude malignancy.

■ If ulcers are severe, atypical, or nonhealing, consider Zollinger-Ellison syndrome (gastrin-secreting tumor).

## Small Bowel Obstruction (SBO)

An SBO results in proximal dilation of intestine due to the accumulation of secretions and air. This condition can result from many causes, but the most common are adhesions, hernias, neoplasms, inflammatory bowel disease, and intussusception. An SBO can be life-threatening if the arterial supply is compromised (strangulated). Patients may present early or late with SBO but usually have intermittent "crampy" pain, copious vomiting, and abdominal distension.

### Pertinent Positives/Negatives: OPQRST

■ **O**nset: sudden or subtle, swallowing of foreign body (dentures)

■ **P**rovocative/**P**alliative: worse with positioning, guarding, eating, or drinking

■ **Q**uality: similar to previous episodes of abdominal pain or previous obstructions

■ **R**egion/**R**adiation: abdominal pain

■ **S**everity: 1 to 10

■ **T**iming: constant or intermittent

Associated features: fever or chills, nausea and vomiting (bilious vs. bloody vs. feculent vs. other), diarrhea or constipation, weight loss, night sweats, appetite or anorexia, melena or hematochezia

Miscellaneous: previous surgeries or radiation therapy, previous episodes of obstruction, last meal, trauma, history of cancer

### Physical Examination

- Fever, hypertension or hypotension, tachycardia
- Abdominal surgical scars; abdominal tenderness (position, peritoneal signs); bowel sounds (hyper "borborygmi" or hypoactive); visible peristalsis; "ladder-like" abdomen; abdominal, inguinal, or femoral hernias
- Rectal examination: blood, mass

### Laboratory Studies

- AAS, CBC, BMP, lactic acid, UA, β-hCG (Fig. 4-3)
- Consider liver function tests, CT, U/S, enteroclysis, barium study (to rule out LBO), surgical intervention

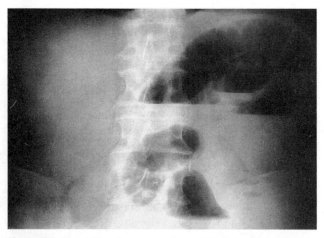

**Figure 4-3** Erect film demonstrating multiple small bowel air-fluid levels. There are multiple air-fluid levels throughout the central portion of the abdomen and numerous dilated loops of small bowel. (*Reproduced with permission from Patel PR. Lecture notes on radiology. Malden, MA: Blackwell Publishing, 1998:110.*)

### 🖊 Management

- ABCs, NPO, correct hypovolemia, NG tube
- Consider antibiotics, surgical intervention if symptoms do not resolve or with development of peritoneal signs

### 🔆 Pearls

- Hyperactive bowel sounds occur early; hypoactive bowel sounds occur late.
- Bilious vomiting is generally an early sign of SBO.
- In children, think of Meckel diverticulum or hernia.
- X-ray findings show dilated loops of small bowel, air-fluid levels on an upright film.
- In very proximal obstruction, bilious vomiting can occur early with minimal distention.
- No reliable way exists to differentiate simple from early strangulated obstruction on physical examination; serial examinations are of utmost importance and can detect changes early.

#### Inflammatory Bowel Disease: A PIE SAC

**A**phthous ulcers
**P**yoderma gangrenosum
**I**ritis
**E**rythema nodosum
**S**clerosing cholangitis
**A**rthritis
**C**lubbing of fingertips

## Spontaneous Bacterial Peritonitis

Spontaneous bacterial peritonitis is an acute bacterial infection of ascitic fluid, usually affecting patients with cirrhosis but also those on peritoneal dialysis, with nephritic syndrome, or with SLE. The pathophysiology of spontaneous bacterial peritonitis is not quite fully understood, but it is likely caused from an impaired immune system with either transmural migration of enteric bacteria or via hematogenous spread. Patients can present asymptomatically, in shock, or can present mimicking an acute surgical abdomen.

## Pertinent Positives/Negatives: OPQRST (see End-Stage Liver Disease/Cirrhosis/Hepatic Encephalopathy)

- **O**nset: sudden onset or subtle onset of symptoms
- **P**rovocative/**P**alliative: not applicable
- **Q**uality: not applicable
- **R**egion/**R**adiation: abdomen
- **S**everity: 1 to 10
- **T**iming: constant or intermittent

Associated features: fever or chills, abdominal pain, increased abdominal girth, worsening ascites, confusion or AMS, diarrhea, change in color or amount of urine

  Miscellaneous: history of liver disease, history of peritoneal dialysis, worsening ascites (refractory to medication), edema

### Physical Examination

- Fever, hypotension, tachycardia or bradycardia
- Abdominal pain, ascites, orthostasis, AMS

### Laboratory Studies

- CBC, CMP with liver enzymes, AAS
- Consider blood cultures, urine cultures, paracentesis for Gram stain, cytology, granulocyte count, pH

## 💊 Management

■ Supportive care, IV antibiotics (ampicillin and an amino-glycoside)

■ Admission

## ✳️ Pearls

■ *Escherichia coli* is the most common organism (50%), followed by *Streptococcus* and *Klebsiella*.

■ Spontaneous bacterial peritonitis can be completely asymptomatic in as many as 30% of patients.

---

## Upper Gastrointestinal Bleeding

Upper GI bleeds are defined as bleeding proximal to the ligament of Treitz (junction of duodenum and jejunum). Patients with upper GI bleeding may present subtly or with a life-threatening condition. There are multiple causes of upper GI bleeding, some relatively benign but some more severe that must be ruled out. Conditions that must be excluded include peptic ulcer disease, gastric erosions, esophageal varices, Mallory-Weiss tears, esophagitis, duodenitis, gastritis, epistaxis, and upper respiratory bleeding.

### Causes of GI Bleeding: ABCDEFGHI

**A**ngiodysplasia

**B**owel cancer

**C**olitis

**D**iverticulitis/ **D**uodenal ulcer

**E**pistaxis/**E**sophageal (cancer, esophagitis, varices)

**F**istula (anal, aortaenteric)

**G**astric (cancer, ulcer, gastritis)

**H**emorrhoids

**I**nfectious diarrhea/ **I**nflammatory bowel disease/ **I**schemic bowel

### Pertinent Positives/Negatives: OPQRST

- **O**nset: sudden or subtle onset of bleeding, previous history of upper GI bleeding or hematemesis
- **P**rovocative/**P**alliative: worse after vomiting or eating
- **Q**uality: gross blood in emesis vs. streaks of blood; quantify but beware of patient's estimate
- **R**egion/**R**adiation: not applicable
- **S**everity: 1 to 10
- **T**iming: constant or intermittent

Associated features: melena or hematochezia, dizziness or lightheadedness, abdominal pain, syncope, chest pain, weakness, AMS, nausea, constipation or diarrhea, hemorrhoids

Miscellaneous: trauma; history of bleeding disorders; alcohol use; liver disease; ascites; ASA, NSAID, or warfarin use; previous surgical history

### Physical Examination

- Hypotension, tachycardia, tachypnea
- Continued bleeding, abdominal pain, AMS, cool skin, diaphoresis, dermatologic manifestations of cirrhosis (telangiectasias, bruises, palmar erythema), ascites
- Rectal examination (Heme positive)
- ENT examination to rule out bleeding due to epistaxis or URI

### Laboratory Studies

- Orthostatic BP, CBC, PT/PTT/INR, type and cross, CMP with LFTs, ECG, UA
- Consider NG tube aspiration (positive for blood), CXR (perforation)

**Management**

■ ABCs, correct hypovolemia, oxygen
■ Consider transfusion, NG tube, IV vasopressin and/or octreotide, endoscopy. In life-threatening bleeding, consider Sengstaken-Blakemore tube.

## Pearls

■ The initial Hct/Hgb may be falsely elevated before it equilibrates after an acute bleed (can take several hours).
■ The BUN may be elevated in GI bleeding because of the GI absorption of RBCs.

 **Literature**

■ Anderson BA, Salem L, Flum DR, et al. A systematic review of whether oral contrast is necessary for the computed tomography of appendicitis in adults. *Am J Surgery*. 2005 Sept:190(3) 474–478. This systematic review identified 23 reports. After analysis, the authors concluded that CT without oral contrast was similar (sensitivity 95% vs. 92%; negative predictive value 96% for both), or surprisingly better (specificity 97% vs. 94%; positive predictive value 97% vs. 89%; accuracy, 96% vs. 92%; P < .0001) than with oral contrast. The authors believe that use of noncontrast CT techniques to diagnose appendicitis showed equivalent or better diagnostic performance compared with CT scanning using oral contrast.
■ Chase CW, Barker DE, Russell WL, et al. Serum amylase and lipase in the evaluation of acute abdominal pain. *Am Surg*. 1996 Dec;62(12):1028–1033. In this article, the authors reported that serum lipase is a better test than serum amylase either to exclude or to support a diagnosis of acute pancreatitis.

- Cheadle WG, Garr EE, Richardson JD. The importance of early diagnosis of small bowel obstruction. *Am Surg.* 1988 Sep;54(9):565–569. In this article, 90% of patients with SBO had at least one prior abdominal procedure; those of a gynecologic or obstetric nature were most common. Abdominal pain (92%), vomiting (82%), abdominal tenderness (64%), and distention (59%) were the most frequent symptoms and signs, and plain abdominal x-rays were abnormal in 273 (91%) patients.

- Chen SC. Nonsurgical management of partial adhesive small-bowel obstruction with oral therapy: a randomized controlled trial. *CMAJ* 2005;173(10):1165–1169. This study reported that oral therapy with magnesium oxide, *Lactobacillus acidophilus*, and simethicone was effective in hastening the resolution of conservatively treated partial adhesive small-bowel obstruction and shortening the hospital stay.

- Corley DA, Stefan AM, Wolf M, et al. Early indicators of prognosis in upper gastrointestinal hemorrhage. *Am J Gastroenterol.* 1998 Mar;93(3):336–340. These results showed five variables to be independent predictors ($p < 0.05$) of an adverse outcome in upper GI bleeding: an initial Hct < 30%, initial SBP < 100 mm Hg, red blood in the NG lavage, history of cirrhosis or ascites on examination, and a history of vomiting red blood.

- Crawford DL, Phillips EH. Laparoscopic repair and groin hernia surgery. *Surg Clin North Am.* 1998 Dec; 78(6): 1047–1062. This article reported that when patients are selected properly and surgeons are adequately trained and proctored, laparoscopic herniorrhaphy can be performed with acceptably low incidences of recurrence and complications as compared to traditional herniorrhaphy techniques.

■ Diehl AK, Sugarek NJ, Todd KH. Clinical evaluation for gallstone disease: usefulness of symptoms and signs in diagnosis. *Am J Med*. 1990 Jul;89(1):29–33. The authors reported that upper abdominal pain is the symptom most closely associated with gallstone disease. Radiation to the upper back, a steady quality, duration between 1 and 24 hours, and onset more than an hour after meals support the diagnosis. Nevertheless, gallstone-associated symptoms are nonspecific, and accurate diagnosis cannot rely on the clinical assessment alone. Careful clinical evaluation can guide patient selection for diagnostic imaging and the appropriate management of people found to harbor stones.

■ Dinis-Ribeiro M, Cortez-Pinto H, Marinho R, et al. Spontaneous bacterial peritonitis in patients with hepatic cirrhosis: evaluation of a treatment protocol at specialized units. *Rev Esp Enferm Dig*. 2002 Aug;94(8): 473–481. The authors reported that renal failure is an important negative prognosis factor in spontaneous bacterial peritonitis.

■ Esses D. Ability of CT to alter decision making in elderly patients with acute abdominal pain. *Am J Emerg Med*. 2004;22(4):270–272. CT changed diagnosis in almost 50% of elderly patients with undifferentiated abdominal pain and changed the disposition in the emergency department in 25% of cases.

■ Kaplan DE, Reddy KR. Rising incidence of hepatocellular carcinoma: the role of hepatitis B and C; the impact on transplantation and outcomes. *Clin Liver Dis*. 2003 Aug;7(3): 683–714. The researchers theorized that after the attrition of older affected generations, the incidence of hepatocellular carcinoma will likely decline rapidly. Although no vaccine is currently available for hepatitis C, Kaplan believes cases are projected to peak and decline because of a marked reduction in transmission as a result of behavioral modification and safeguarding of blood supplies.

■ Lee SL, Walsh AJ, Ho HS. Computed tomography and ultrasonography do not improve and may delay the diagnosis and treatment of acute appendicitis. *Arch Surg.* 2001;36:556–562. Neither CT nor U/S improved the diagnostic accuracy or the negative appendectomy rate and may actually delay consultation and appendectomy.

■ Megraud F, on behalf of the European Pediatric Task Force on *Helicobacter pylori*. Comparison of non-invasive tests to detect *Helicobacter pylori* infection in children and adolescents: results of a multicenter European study. *J Pediatr.* 2005;146:198–203. Fecal antigen testing for *H. pylori* is safe and very sensitive. However, recent reports show the urease breath test may be more accurate.

■ Ong JP, Aggarwal A, Krieger D, et al. Correlation between ammonia levels and the severity of hepatic encephalopathy. *Am J Med.* 2003 Feb 15;114(3):188–193. Ammonia levels correlate with the severity of hepatic encephalopathy (contrary to popular belief). Venous sampling is adequate for ammonia measurement.

■ Santander C, Gravalos RG, Gomez-Cedenilla A, et al. Antimicrobial therapy for *Helicobacter pylori* infection versus long-term maintenance antisecretion treatment in the prevention of recurrent hemorrhage from peptic ulcer: prospective nonrandomized trial on 125 patients. *Am J Gastroenterol.* 1996 Aug;91(8):1549–1552. The researchers reported that cure of *H. pylori* infection reduces the recurrence of peptic ulcer and of rebleeding from ulcer disease more effectively than long-term maintenance therapy.

■ Spiegel BM, Ofman JJ, Woods K, et al. Minimizing recurrent peptic ulcer hemorrhage after endoscopic hemostasis: the cost-effectiveness of competing strategies. *Am J Gastroenterol.* 2003;98(1):86–97. IV pantoprazole (Protonix) significantly improved outcomes and decreased hospital costs in the setting of upper GI bleeding.

■ Vriens PW. Computed tomography severity index is an early prognostic tool for acute pancreatitis. *J Am Coll Surg.* 2005;201(4):497–502. CT severity index on initial CT at diagnosis more accurately predicts pancreatitis prognosis than Ranson's criteria.

# Hematology System

## Anemia

Anemia is the presence of a decreased number of circulating RBCs, resulting in a low Hgb/Hct relative to baseline values (usually <12 mg/dL in women; <14 mg/dL in men). There are multiple causes of anemia, but initially anemia should be divided into two categories, emergent and nonemergent. The differential diagnosis of anemia includes the following conditions: iron deficiency, post-traumatic, kidney disease, vitamin deficiency, pregnancy, alcoholism, SCA, hemolytic anemia, thalassemia, liver disease, cancer, hypothyroidism, chemotherapy, GI bleeding, menstrual losses, bone marrow disorders, SLE, anemia of chronic disease, aplastic anemia, medications, splenomegaly, and laboratory error.

It may be helpful to view anemia as either the destruction of RBCs, decreased RBC production, or blood loss. Depending on whether the anemia is chronic or acute, the patient may be symptomatic or completely asymptomatic. The types of anemia are listed in Table 5-1.

### Pertinent Positives/Negatives: OPQRST

- **O**nset: length of time patient has been anemic, history of anemia, past workup for anemia, when symptoms began
- **P**rovocative/**P**alliative: not applicable
- **Q**uality: any dyspnea on exertion, lightheadedness on standing?
- **R**egion/**R**adiation: not applicable

**TABLE 5-1**

## Types of Anemia

Macrocytic Anemia (implies red blood cell maturation defect)
    Vitamin $B_{12}$ deficiency
    Folic acid deficiency
    Alcohol abuse
    Liver disease
    Marrow aplasia
    Myelofibrosis
    Reticulocytosis
    Hypothyroidism

Microcytic (implies abnormal hemoglobin synthesis)
    Iron deficiency anemia
    Thalassemia
    Hemoglobinopathy
    Anemia of chronic disease
    Sideroblastic anemia
    Chronic renal failure
    Lead poisoning

■ **S**everity: not applicable

■ **T**iming: constant or intermittent

Miscellaneous: history of anemia or low blood count; trauma; bleeding; orthostatic vital signs but also orthostatic symptoms (dizziness on standing); thirst; AMS; decreased urine; easy bruising; hematemesis, melena, or hematochezia; hemoptysis; heavy or frequent menses; medications; recent surgeries; recent travel; family history of anemia or blood disorder; weakness; fatigue; dyspnea; chest pain; tachycardia; syncope; weight loss; night sweats; cancer; back pain; jaundice; spontaneous purpura; pregnancies; hematuria; poor nutrition; pica (urge to eat clay or ice chips)

## Physical Examination

- Fever, hypotension, tachycardia, tachypnea, orthostatic BP, narrow pulse pressure, AMS, pallor (skin/conjunctiva), diaphoresis, bruises/petechiae/purpura, jaundice, evidence of bleeding, systolic flow murmur, peripheral pulses, abdominal pain, hepatosplenomegaly, abdominal masses
- Rectal examination with stool guaiac
- Pelvic examination if vaginal bleeding
- Neurological examination for altered position/vibratory sense

## Laboratory Studies

- CBC with RBC indices (MCV, MCH), CMP, reticulocyte count, peripheral blood smear, iron studies, bilirubin, LDH, haptoglobin, blood type and screen
- Consider endoscopy, bone marrow biopsy

## Management

- Treat the underlying disease.
- Consider blood transfusion at Hgb less than 8.5 g/dL if there are no contraindications.

## Pearls

- Macrocytic anemia (MCV > 100 fL): vitamin $B_{12}$/folate deficiency, hemolytic anemia, alcohol use, liver disease
- Microcytic anemia (MCV < 100 fL): iron deficiency anemia, anemia of chronic disease, thalassemia
- Normocytic anemia: hemorrhage, hemolysis, infection, any cause of microcytic or macrocytic anemia
- A sharp increase in BUN may indicate a GI bleed.
- Acute bleeding may not lower the Hgb/Hct for several hours until equilibration occurs.

## Disseminated Intravascular Coagulation (DIC)

DIC is a complex acquired coagulopathy that involves intravascular fibrin and the consumption of procoagulants and platelets. Predisposing conditions include trauma, infection, sepsis, obstetrical complications, and severe transfusion reaction. DIC should be suspected in any patient who develops purpura; bleeding; and signs of injury to organs, especially the CNS or kidney. In DIC, tissue factor, thrombin, and plasmin are systemically circulated, resulting in coagulation (causing thrombotic injury) and the exhaustion of the factors of coagulation. This leads to coagulopathy.

### Pertinent Positives/Negatives: OPQRST

■ **O**nset: when symptoms began

■ **P**rovocative/**P**alliative: not applicable

■ **Q**uality: not applicable

■ **R**egion/**R**adiation: possible back, joint, or abdominal pain

■ **S**everity: not applicable

■ **T**iming: constant or intermittent

Miscellaneous: bleeding (epistaxis, gingival/mucosal bleeding), fevers, recent trauma, AMS, dizziness, fatigue, weakness, medications, cancer, weight loss, night sweats, recent transfusion, burns, head injury, pregnancy, recent delivery, vaginal bleeding, snake bites, shunts

###  Physical Examination

■ Fever, tachycardia or bradycardia, hypertension or hypotension, orthostatic vital signs (decreased), evidence of bleeding from any organ system, evidence of thrombosis (acral cyanosis, skin necrosis)

■ Pelvic examination (evidence of infection, retained products of conception, foreign body)

### 🔬 Laboratory Studies (Fig. 5-1)

■ CBC with platelet count, PT/PTT/INR, thrombin time, fibrinogen level, D-dimer, UA

■ Consider additional tests for specific etiology

### 💊 Management

■ ABCs

■ Treat the underlying disorder

■ Replace platelets/cryoprecipitate/fresh frozen plasma

■ Give antibiotics if indicated

■ Consider heparin/antithrombin III

### ✳ Pearls

■ PT/PTT/INR: prolonged

■ D-dimer: high

■ Platelets and Hgb: low

---

## Sickle Cell Anemia

SCA is an autosomal recessive disorder resulting in hemoglobin S in RBCs. It is formed by the substitution of valine for glutamine in the β hemoglobin chain. This results in a "sickled" RBC that is less deformable in the capillary beds, resulting in sludging of the blood. This leads to vaso-occlusive and thrombotic events, chronic hemolysis, infectious crises, and organ injury.

### Pertinent Positives/Negatives: OPQRST

■ **O**nset: when current symptoms began

■ **P**rovocative/**P**alliative: consider conditions that make SCA worse (e.g., stress, weather, concomitant illness,

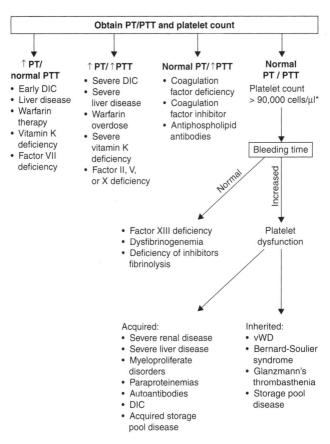

| Obtain PT/PTT and platelet count |
|---|

**↑ PT/ normal PTT**
- Early DIC
- Liver disease
- Warfarin therapy
- Vitamin K deficiency
- Factor VII deficiency

**↑ PT/ ↑PTT**
- Severe DIC
- Severe liver disease
- Warfarin overdose
- Severe vitamin K deficiency
- Factor II, V, or X deficiency

**Normal PT/ ↑PTT**
- Coagulation factor deficiency
- Coagulation factor inhibitor
- Antiphospholipid antibodies

**Normal PT / PTT**
Platelet count > 90,000 cells/μl*

| Bleeding time |
|---|

*Normal* / *Increased*

- Factor XIII deficiency
- Dysfibrinogenemia
- Deficiency of inhibitors fibrinolysis

Platelet dysfunction

Acquired:
- Severe renal disease
- Severe liver disease
- Myeloproliferate disorders
- Paraproteinemias
- Autoantibodies
- DIC
- Acquired storage pool disease

Inherited:
- vWD
- Bernard-Soulier syndrome
- Glanzmann's thrombasthenia
- Storage pool disease

*A platelet count less than 90,000 cells/μl may result in an increased bleeding time and a bleeding disorder. Patients with platelet counts greater than 90,000 cells/μl may still be thrombocytopenic (i.e., a platelet count less than 15,000 cells/μl), but this level of thrombocytopenia is usually not the cause of a bleeding disorder; therefore, other causes should be considered.

**Figure 5-1** Approach to the patient with a bleeding disorder. DIC = disseminated intravascular coagulation; PT = prothrombin time; PTT = partial thromboplastin time; vWD = von Willebrand disease. (*From Saint S and Frances C. Saint Frances Guide to Inpatient Medicine. Philadelphia: Lippincott Williams & Wilkins, 1997:334.*)

medications) or better, consider what medications ame-
liorate the SCA pain

- **Q**uality: ask the patient to describe his or her current
  pain and whether it is similar to previous exacerbations
  of SCA
- **R**egion/**R**adiation: possible headache; possible neck, back,
  abdominal, chest pain, joint/bone, or back pain
- **S**everity: consider the severity of the SCA and whether the
  patient has the disease or trait
- **T**iming: constant or intermittent

Miscellaneous: history and family history of SCA; syncope;
preceding infection or URI; previous episodes of pain; alcohol use; recent air travel; exposure to cold; exercise; dyspnea;
visual blurring; AMS; jaundice; pallor; fatigue; fevers or
chills, history of splenectomy, vaccines, abdominal surgeries;
hematuria; priapism; urinary symptoms; weakness or aphasia; analgesic use; pregnancy; emotional stress

###  Physical Examination (Table 5-2)

- Fever, tachycardia or bradycardia, hypertension or hypotension, orthostatic vital signs
- Examine for *any* sign of local infection, jaundice, scleral
  icterus, pallor, AMS, nuchal rigidity, evidence of CHF, $S_3/S_4$,
  rales/rhonchi/consolidation, abdominal tenderness/radia-
  tion, hepatomegaly, splenomegaly, presence of surgical
  scars, priapism, focal neurologic deficits

### Laboratory Studies

- CBC (compare with previous tests), CMP, reticulocyte
  count, peripheral blood smear, UA, β-hCG, CXR
- Consider ABG, ECG, AAS, Hgb electrophoresis, bone scan

**TABLE 5-2**

## Clinical Manifestations of Sickle Cell Anemia

| Related to Chronic Hemolytic Anemia | Related to Abnormal Adhesions, Sickling, and Vaso-occlusion | Related to Increased Susceptibility to Infection |
|---|---|---|
| Normocytic anemia | Painful crises | Pneumococcal sepsis |
| Elevated bilirubin and LDH | Cerebrovascular accident | *Salmonella* sepsis |
| Gallstone disease | Acute and chronic cardiopulmonary disease (e.g., acute chest syndromes, cor pulmonale) | Osteomyelitis |
| | Priapism | |
| | Splenic autoinfarction | |
| | Skeletal changes (e.g., aseptic necrosis of the hip) | |

(From Myers AR [ed.]. NMS Medicine, 5th ed Philadelphia: Lippincott Williams & Wilkins. 2005:125.)

 **Management**

■ Correct hypovolemia/rehydrate, give oxygen, and administer analgesia (mainstays of treatment for vaso-occlusive attacks).

■ Consider transfusion.

■ Treat infection with appropriate antibiotics.

**Sickle Cell Complications: SICKLE**

**S**trokes/**S**welling of hands and feet/**S**pleen problems
**I**nfections/ **I**nfarctions

**C**rises (painful, sequestration, aplastic)/**C**holelithiasis/**C**hest syndrome/
**C**hronic hemolysis/**C**ardiac problems
**K**idney disease
**L**iver disease/**L**ung problems
**E**rection (priapism)/**E**ye problems (retinopathy)

## ❈ Pearls

■ Most patients with SCA have a baseline anemia, but a major
drop in hemoglobin (e.g., more than 2 g/dL) from previously recorded values indicates a hematological crisis.

■ Leukocytosis is expected in all patients with SCA. Major
elevation in the WBC count (i.e., >20,000/mm$^3$) with a left
shift raises suspicion for infection.

---

## Thrombotic Thrombocytopenic Purpura (TTP)
## and Idiopathic Thrombocytopenic Purpura (ITP)

TTP and ITP are two clinical entities that are often confused but
are clinically distinct. TTP is classically seen as thrombocytopenic purpura, fever, renal dysfunction, neurologic
abnormalities, and microangiopathic hemolytic anemia, and
is the result of subendothelial deposits of fibrin and platelet
aggregates in the vasculature. ITP is an autoimmune platelet
disorder resulting in increased peripheral destruction of
platelets that leads to mucosal bleeding, purpura, and easy
bruising.

### Pertinent Positives/Negatives: OPQRST

■ **O**nset: time that symptoms began, possible history of symptoms, possible previous diagnosis of bleeding problem

■ **P**rovocative/**P**alliative: consider conditions that make symptoms worse or better

■ **Q**uality: not applicable
■ **R**egion/**R**adiation: not applicable
■ **S**everity: not applicable
■ **T**iming: constant or intermittent

Miscellaneous: fever or chills, recent viral infection, medications (especially heparin, ranitidine), risk factors for HIV, pregnancy, history of cancer, night sweats, weight loss, drug or alcohol use, bleeding (type, severity, previous episodes, family history), bruising tendency, menorrhagia, hematuria, chest discomfort, weakness, fatigue, AMS, headaches, neurologic symptoms (seizures, hemiparesis), arthralgias, abdominal pain, recent immunizations

 **Physical Examination**
■ Fever, tachycardia or bradycardia, hypertension or hypotension, orthostatic vital signs
■ AMS, rash, petechiae/purpura/ecchymosis, bruising, evidence of bleeding (especially mucosal/epistaxis), vaginal bleeding, jaundice, pallor, neurologic symptoms, CVA tenderness, splenomegaly

 **Laboratory Studies (Fig. 5-1)**
■ CBC with differential, CMP, β-hCG, UA, PT/PTT/INR, bleeding time, peripheral blood smear
■ Consider LDH, indirect bilirubin, fibrinogen, D-dimer, HIV testing, head CT

 **Management**
■ TTP
    ■ Plasmapheresis, corticosteroids, aspirin
    ■ Consider splenectomy

- ITP
  - Pediatric patients resolve spontaneously
  - Adults may require corticosteroids, IVIG
  - Consider splenectomy

## ✷ Pearls

- TTP is a clinical diagnosis.
- Splenomegaly is present in TTP, not ITP.
- Hemolytic-uremic syndrome is TTP without the fever and neurologic deficits.

## 📖 Literature

- Corwin HL, Surgenor SD, Gettinger A. Transfusion practice in the critically ill. *Crit Care Med*. 2003 Dec;31(12 Suppl):S668–671. The authors wrote that most critically ill patients can tolerate Hgb levels as low as 7 mg/dL.

- Levi M, de Jonge E, van der Poll T, et al. Novel approaches to the management of disseminated intravascular coagulation. *Crit Care Med*. 2000 Sep;28(9 Suppl): S20–S24. "Although the cornerstone of DIC management is the specific and vigorous treatment of the underlying disorder, strategies aimed at inhibiting coagulation activation may theoretically be justified. Such strategies have been found to be beneficial in experimental and initial clinical studies. These strategies, which follow from our current understanding of the pathophysiology of DIC, involve inhibition of tissue factor-mediated activation of coagulation or restoration of physiologic anticoagulant pathways by means of the administration of antithrombin concentrate or (activated) protein C concentrate. Although no complete evidence from controlled clinical trials is available for most of the proposed therapeutic interventions, these novel strategies are being studied."

■ Medina PJ, Sipols JM, George JN. Drug-associated thrombotic thrombocytopenic purpura-hemolytic uremic syndrome. *Curr Opin Hematol*. 2001 Sep;8(5):286–293. Five drugs that have been the subject of the most recent reports of drug-associated TTP–hemolytic-uremic syndrome are discussed: mitomycin C, cyclosporine, quinine, ticlopidine, and clopidogrel.

■ Vichinsky EP, Neumayr LD, Earles AN, et al. Causes and outcomes of the acute chest syndrome in sickle cell disease. National Acute Chest Syndrome Study Group. *N Engl J Med*. 2000 Jun 22;342(25):1855–1865. The authors wrote "In patients with sickle cell disease, the acute chest syndrome is commonly precipitated by fat embolism and infection, especially community-acquired pneumonia. Among older patients and those with neurologic symptoms, the syndrome often progresses to respiratory failure. Treatment with transfusions and bronchodilators improves oxygenation, and with aggressive treatment, most patients who have respiratory failure recover."

# 6 Obstetrics and Gynecology

## Initial Evaluation of the Pregnant Patient

### Pertinent Positives/Negatives

- Obstetric history (gravida, para), estimated date of confinement, IUP by LMP and/or U/S
- Prenatal care, pregnancy complications, vaginal bleeding (amount), contractions (frequency and duration), loss of fluid/rupture of membranes
- Positive fetal movement
- Back pain, pelvic pressure

### Physical Examination

- Fever, abdominal tenderness, CVA tenderness
- Sterile speculum examination: cervical dilation, pooling
- Sterile vaginal examination only if there is placenta previa or preterm premature rupture of membranes
- Lower extremity edema/pain/tenderness, vaginal bleeding plus FHTs/variability/acceleration/deceleration

### Laboratory Studies

- Urine dip for protein, ± nitrazine, ferning on smear, type plus Rh, reassuring FHTs, cervical dilation
- U/S (may show vertex/malpresentation/cervical dilation/placenta previa/oligohydramnios)

## ❁ Pearls

- Nitrazine test for pH of vagina: amniotic fluid is more basic; therefore, the color of the nitrazine changes from yellow to blue in a more basic environment. False-positive results are caused by contamination of semen, blood, or infection.

- Ferning: Smear from posterior fornix of vagina is allowed to dry and examined under a microscope. A "ferning" pattern is seen in the presence of ruptured membranes. (Be aware that cervical mucus can cause ferning, which looks more like palm fronds.)

- Vaginal pooling: fluid collection in the posterior fornix of vagina may be amniotic fluid.

## Evaluation of the Fetus

Four questions that should be asked of all pregnant patients are:

1. Do you have any vaginal bleeding?
2. Have you experienced any loss of fluids?
3. Are you experiencing any fetal movement?
4. Are you having any contractions?

## ✐ Physical Examination

- Fundal height: measure from the pubic symphysis to the top of the fundus in centimeters

- This number ±3 cm is the approximate fetal age in weeks (Fig. 6-1)

## ❁ Pearls

- FHTs should be checked by Doppler U/S at 10–12 weeks
- Fetal movement (quickening) usually between 16 and 20 weeks

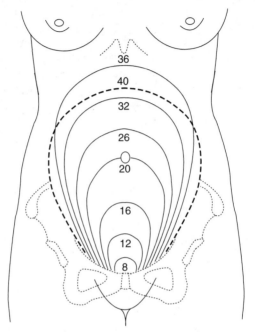

**Figure 6-1** Fundal measurement and number of weeks' gestation. (*After Scott JR, DiSaia PJ, Hammond CB, et al. (eds) Danforth's Obstetrics and Gynecology, 6th ed. Philadelphia: J.B. Lippincott, 1990: 135.*)

## Preeclampsia/Eclampsia (Pregnancy-Induced Hypertension)

Preeclampsia/eclampsia is encountered in 6%–8% of all pregnancies and is a significant cause of maternal mortality (10%–12%). It usually occurs before labor but can also occur in the intrapartum/postpartum period. Vasospasm is the main component and affects multiple organ systems. The three signs and symptoms that form the classic triad of preeclampsia are edema, hypertension, and proteinuria. However, 10% of normal gravid women have edema of the face and/or hands. Risk factors for preeclampsia include previous preeclampsia, primiparity, multifetal gestation, chronic hypertension, pregestational DM, antiphospholipid antibody deficiency syndrome, obesity, age greater than 35 years, and African-American race.

Eclampsia is preeclampsia with CNS involvement (seizures). Eclampsia is considered a true emergency, and delivery should be considered once the patient is stabilized (taking gestational age into account). Preeclampsia is associated with an increased risk of placental abruption. After eclamptic seizures, a head CT is recommended to ensure that no resultant damage occurred or to rule out intracranial causes of seizures.

## Pertinent Positives/Negatives

■ Headache, edema (face and hands), weight gain, blurred vision

■ Epigastric pain (distention of liver capsule), nausea/vomiting

### Physical Examination

■ Hypertension (140/90 mm Hg or MAP > 105 mm Hg)

■ Hyperactive reflexes/clonus, tender RUQ, generalized edema

### Laboratory Studies

■ Proteinuria (3 or 4 on urine protein dipstick or >0.3 g/L in 24-hour urine collection), elevated serum BUN and Cr, elevated uric acid

■ Thrombocytopenia and decreased serum fibrinogen, elevated AST/ALT, increased PT/PTT

## 🔲 Management

- Delivery/expected management
  - Mild preeclampsia: expectant management until full term or unless becomes severe preeclampsia
  - Severe preeclampsia: delivery versus observation in hospital
  - Severe preeclampsia plus HELLP: delivery no matter the gestation
- Prophylactic management should be given to all patients with preeclampsia.
  - Magnesium sulfate is the most commonly used agent.
  - Toxic levels of magnesium sulfate lead to respiratory depression, respiratory arrest, and cardiac arrest. Stop magnesium infusion and give calcium gluconate.
- Eclampsia is treated with magnesium, benzodiazepines, phenytoin, and pentobarbital. Hypertension can be managed with labetalol or hydralazine.

## ❊ Pearls

- HELLP can occur in up to 20% of women with severe preeclampsia; they do not necessarily have proteinuria.
- Diagnosis of severe preeclampsia (need only one):
  - SBP >160 mm Hg or DBP >110 mm Hg on two occasions 6 hours apart while on bed rest
  - Proteinuria (5 g in 24-hour urine or 3+/4 on two occasions 4 hours apart)
  - Oliguria (<500 mL in 24 hours)
  - Cerebral or visual disturbances (headache)
  - Pulmonary edema or cyanosis
  - RUQ pain
  - Elevated liver function tests

- Thrombocytopenia
- Intrauterine growth restriction

■ Patients with chronic hypertension may develop superimposed preeclampsia (increased proteinuria after 20 weeks gestation, compared to earlier baseline 24-hour urine).

■ Headaches and hyperactive reflexes are absent in up to 20% of patients who develop eclampsia.

■ Gestational hypertension is elevated BP after 20 weeks gestation but without proteinuria; BP returns to normal postpartum. Twenty-five percent of patients with gestational hypertension develop preeclampsia.

## Vaginal Bleeding (First Half of Pregnancy)

Presence or absence of pregnancy should be confirmed via urine hCG or serum hCG. If the woman is in the first half of pregnancy, spontaneous abortion (loss of pregnancy before 20 weeks), ectopic pregnancy, trophoblastic disease, implantation bleeding, and infection should be considered (Table 6-1).

### Pertinent Positives/Negatives

■ LMP, amount of bleeding (number of pads per day), blood type, abdominal/vaginal pain

■ Syncope, dizziness/orthostatic symptoms

■ Fever, uterine contractions, previous episodes, previous miscarriages, history of bleeding dyscrasias, recent intercourse, shoulder pain

### 🖉 Physical Examination

■ Orthostatic BP, fever

■ Cervical dilation, presence of tissue, confirmation of bleeding, CMT, adnexal masses/tenderness, tender uterus

---

### TABLE 6-1

## Classification of Spontaneous Abortions

**Types**

- Threatened: pregnancy-related bloody discharge during first half of pregnancy without cervical dilation
- Inevitable: cervical dilation combined with vaginal bleeding
- Incomplete: Passage of parts of products of conception (os open with bleeding)
- Complete: passage of all tissue (os usually closed with minimal or no bleeding)
- Missed: fetal death without passage of any tissue (± spotting, cervix closed)
- Septic: evidence of infection during any stage of abortion

**Diagnosis and Treatment**

- Depending on the type of abortion, serum β-hCG, U/S (to confirm IUP, absence of FHT), D&C/evacuation of pregnancy, antibiotics if septic
- Outpatient workup if history of multiple spontaneous abortions

---

### 🔬 Laboratory Studies

- CBC, blood type, Rh factor/antibody screen, UA, serum β-hCG
- Transabdominal/transvaginal U/S

### 💊 Management

- Assess cervix
- Correct for hypotension, evaluate for surgical emergency (ectopic pregnancy)
- If unsensitized, give RhoGAM

# 🎴 Pearls

■ With β-hCG level greater than 1500 IU/mL, a gestational sac can be seen on transvaginal U/S. After the LMP, the yolk sac is seen at 5 weeks, and the heart beat is heard between 6 and 7 weeks.

■ With a normal IUP, the β-hCG should approximately double (increase by at least >66%) every 2 days.

## Vaginal Bleeding (Second Half of Pregnancy)

Pregnancy should be confirmed via urine β-hCG and physical examination.

### Pertinent Positives/Negatives

■ Pain, rupture of membranes, positive fetal movement, vaginal discharge, amount of bleeding, passage of tissue, fevers, recent intercourse, contractions

■ Trauma, cocaine use

■ Previous cesarean sections, previous history of preterm labor

### 📓 Physical Examination

■ Abdominal pain, tender uterus, vaginal bleeding

■ *Digital and speculum examination should be avoided if considering placenta previa* (Table 6-2)

■ Confirm reassuring FHTs

### 🔬 Laboratory Studies

■ CBC, type and cross, PT/PTT/INR, BUN/Cr, fibrinogen levels

---

### TABLE 6-2

## Abruptio Placentae versus Placenta Previa

**Abruptio placentae: premature separation of the implanted placenta from the uterine wall**

- True obstetric emergency; emergent obstetrical consultation required for monitoring/delivery. Rh isoimmunization prophylaxis may be needed.
- Presenting symptoms: sudden onset of vaginal bleeding, tender uterus, uterine contractions/irritability
- Can be spontaneous (hypertension) or induced (trauma/cocaine)
- U/S: allows exclusion of placenta previa but may not show abruptio placentae

**Placenta Previa: implantation of placenta over the cervical os**

- Incidence increased with multiparity, previous placenta previa, prior cesarean section
- Characteristics: painless vaginal bleeding, nontender uterus
- U/S: confirms placental placement (93%–98% sensitive)
- No pelvic/cervical examination (can precipitate tremendous vaginal bleeding), unless patient in OR prepped for emergent cesarean section

---

### 🔖 Management

- Be aware of DIC in abruptio placentae. Emergent delivery may be necessary if the abruption is severe (see Table 6-2).
- Restore intravascular volume

### 🎴 Pearls

- Placenta previa: painless vaginal bleeding in pregnancy
- Abruptio placentae: painful vaginal bleeding in pregnancy
- "Bloody show": passage of small amount of blood mixed with mucus at the onset of labor

## Ectopic Pregnancy

An ectopic pregnancy is any pregnancy outside the uterine cavity. The classic presentation is abdominal pain with vaginal bleeding in a woman with amenorrhea. Presence should be confirmed by urine β-hCG. Figure 6-2 shows sites of ectopic pregnancies. Diagnoses that should be considered as well as ectopic pregnancy include miscarriage, implantation bleeding, PID, molar pregnancy, and GI disease. Alternative diagnoses for abdominal pain with vaginal bleeding include miscarriage, implantation bleeding, PID, molar pregnancy, and GI disease. Risk factors include tubal surgeries, history of PID, previous ectopic pregnancies, IUDs, and assisted reproductive techniques.

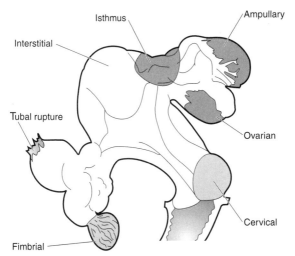

**Figure 6-2** Sites of ectopic pregnancies. (*From Callahan T and Caughey A. Blueprints Obstetrics and Gynecology, 4th ed. Philadelphia: Lippincott Williams & Wilkins , 2007:12.*)

**Pertinent Positives/Negatives**

▪ Abdominal pain, orthostatic symptoms/hypovolemia, shoulder pain

▪ Amenorrhea, first date of LMP, vaginal bleeding

### 🔧 Physical Examination

▪ Fever, orthostatic BP

▪ Peritoneal signs, adnexal mass/tenderness, CMT, blood in vaginal vault, uterine size

### 🔬 Laboratory Studies

▪ Urine/serum β-hCG, immediate U/S, progesterone, CBC, type and Rh

▪ Culdocentesis

### 💊 Management

▪ Evaluate for emergent surgery

▪ Consider expectant versus surgical versus medical treatment

▪ Correct hypovolemia, give RhoGAM

### ✳ Pearls

▪ All women with abdominal pain require a β-hCG.

▪ An IUP can be visualized by transvaginal U/S at β-hCG >1500 IU/mL (5 weeks) (transabdominal U/S at β-hCG >6500 IU/mL).

▪ Beware a heterotopic pregnancy (incidence of 1/30,000)

▪ With a normal IUP, the β-hCG should approximately double (increase by at least >66%) every two days.

▪ A pseudosac is seen in ectopic pregnancies; it is irregularly shaped, blood-filled, and has no yolk sac.

## Pregestational/Gestational Diabetes

Gestational diabetes occurs in up to 5% of all pregnancies. It can result in fetal deformity (especially renal), neonatal hypoglycemia, macrosomia, and shoulder dystocia.

### Pertinent Positives/Negatives
- History of gestational diabetes, history of macrosomic (large) infants, history of miscarriages/stillbirths, history of diabetes, family history of diabetes
- Obesity, polyuria, polydipsia, recurrent yeast infections/ UTIs

 ### Laboratory Studies
- UA, $HgbA_{1c}$, GTT

 ### Management
- Diet, insulin
- Monitor fetal growth and amniotic fluid index
- Consider delivery by cesarean section if neonate weighs >4500 g
- Begin nonstress tests after 32 weeks, depending on severity

### Pearls
- Abnormal GTT (performed 24–28 weeks gestation), showing fasting hyperglycemia >105 mg/dL (Table 6-3)
- GTT at 1 hour (>140 mg/dL) should be followed by 3-hour GTT.
- Many patients develop type 2 DM later in life.

### TABLE 6-3

## Types of Glucose Tolerance Tests

**Carpenter/Coustan Classification**

- Fasting: 95 mg/dL
- 1 hour: 180 mg/dL
- 2 hour: 155 mg/dL
- 3 hour: 140 mg/dL

**National Diabetes Data Group**

- Fasting: 105 mg/dL
- 1 hour: 190 mg/dL
- 2 hour: 165 mg/dL

## Normal Labor

Labor is defined as the progressive effacement and dilation of the cervix in the presence of uterine contractions (<5 minutes apart). Be aware of "false" labor (Braxton Hicks contractions with no dilation/effacement that occur in the last 4 to 8 weeks of pregnancy).

- First stage of labor
    - Latent: cervix dilates to 4 cm and effaces, regular contractions
    - Active: 4 cm–10 cm, regular intense contractions, fetal head descends
- Second stage of labor: complete dilation and delivery of infant
- Third stage of labor: delivery of infant and placenta

## Indications for Cesarean Section

■ Cephalopelvic disproportion, placenta previa, abruptio placentae, fetal malposition, nonreassuring FHTs or fetal distress, prolapsed cord, arrested second stage of labor

■ Active herpetic infection within 2 weeks of delivery, maternal demise

## ❊ Pearls

■ Episiotomy:
   ■ First degree: involves mucosa and skin only
   ■ Second degree: involves skin and muscle
   ■ Third degree: involves skin, muscle, and anal sphincter
   ■ Fourth degree: involves skin, muscle, anal sphincter, and anal wall

■ First stage of labor is shorter in multiparas than in nulliparas.

## Premature Rupture of Membranes (Rupture of Fetal Membranes before Labor Begins)

■ Diagnose with pooling/nitrazine/ferning

■ Increases risk of chorioamnionitis

■ If fetus >37 weeks, consider delivery within 24 hours.

## Preterm Labor (20–37 Weeks Gestation)

■ Consider glucocorticoids to aid fetal lung maturity, tocolysis (magnesium, terbutaline, nifedipine)

■ Cervical length measurements (>35 mm after 24 weeks is desired)

■ Fetal fibronectin after 22 weeks: test that determines likelihood of preterm delivery in patients with contractions
   ■ Fetal fibronectin is normally found in fetal membranes.

- The test is performed by sterile speculum examination and swabbing the posterior vaginal fornix.
- If the fetal fibronectin is negative, then the chance of not delivering in the next 2 weeks is 95%.

## Abnormal Labor

Abnormal labor may occur because of noncephalic or asynclitic presentations, arrested descent, or maternal fatigue. Delivery by forceps or vacuum extractor should be considered.

### Shoulder Dystocia

- Obstetric emergency that occurs when the anterior shoulder is delayed in delivery
- Incidence: 0.6%–1.4%; it is more likely in a macrosomic fetus.
- Fetal asphyxia is a major complication
  - Immediately call for help, perform the McRoberts maneuver, apply suprapubic pressure, rotate the shoulders, perform an episiotomy/proctoepisiotomy, and deliver posterior arm.
  - Consider fracture of clavicle/Zavanelli maneuver.
- Severe dystocias can result in asphyxia and death.

### Nuchal Cord

- Immediately unwrap and loosen cord; if unable, clamp, and cut once shoulder has been delivered.
- Never apply fundal pressure!

### Pearls

- "Turtle" sign: recoil of the fetal chin into perineum immediately after delivery of head

- McRoberts maneuver: sharp flexion of the hips so that the knees are brought to the patient's chest
- Zavanelli maneuver: terbutaline is given, the fetus is pushed back into the vagina, and the fetus is delivered via cesarean section (considered *only* in catastrophic cases)
- Frank breech: flexion of legs at hips but extension at knees
- Footling breech: extension of one or both legs at hips so that knees or feet are presenting
- Complete breech: flexion of both thighs and knees
- Neonatal injuries: brachial plexus, facial bruising, fracture of clavicle or humerus; most resolve without sequelae

## Postpartum Hemorrhage

Such hemorrhage may occur early (in first 24 hours postpartum) or late (24 hours to 6 weeks postpartum). Blood loss is more than 500 mL after vaginal delivery or more than 1000 mL after cesarean delivery. Uterine atony, vaginal/cervical/rectal lacerations, retained products of conception, inverted uterus, coagulopathy, and uterine rupture should be considered.

###  Physical Examination
- Fever
- Palpate uterus for softness, hematomas, masses, "bogginess," retained tissues

###  Laboratory Studies
- Consider CBC, PT/PTT, fibrinogen, fibrin split products, type and cross

### 💊 Management

- Correct blood loss/hypovolemia with IV fluids/PRBCs, $O_2$
- Initially massage uterine fundus and give oxytocin
- Repair any lacerations if any
- Remove any retained products of conception
- If there is no response, consider methylergonovine (Methergine) (contraindicated in hypertensives), carboprost tromethamine (Hemabate) (contraindicated in asthmatics), or prostaglandin $E_2$; consider surgical management

### ❇️ Pearls

- The most common cause of postpartum hemorrhage is uterine atony (>90%).
- Risks factors for uterine atony: macrosomia, multifetal gestations, prolonged labor, induction with oxytocin, polyhydramnios, chorioamnionitis

---

## Evaluation of the Postpartum Patient (Table 6-4)

### Regular Gynecologic Examination

#### Pertinent Positives/Negatives

- Pertinent history: menses (regularity/duration/dysmenorrhea)
- Vaginal discharge, desires for contraception vs. conception, pelvic pain (cyclic/noncyclic), dyspareunia

### 📔 Physical Examination

- Vital signs, hCG urine dipstick, weight, LMP
- General examination (many women use their obstetrician/gynecologists as their primary care physician)

### TABLE 6-4
## Evaluation of the Postpartum Patient

**Normal conditions at postpartum visit**

- Almost normal size of uterus at 6 weeks
- Healed episiotomy site/cesarean section site
- Minimal to no lochia alba
- Possible return of normal menses

**Topics to address**

- Birth control method
- Need for annual Pap smear
- Adaptation of mother to the role of parenthood

**Problems at postpartum visit**

- Fever: rule out endometritis, episiotomy/cesarean section infections or hematomas, mastitis, breast abscess, septic pelvic thrombophlebitis
- Bleeding: rule out retained placenta, damaged episiotomy site, hemorrhoids
- Depression: assess social support, partner support, may need antidepressants if mild, immediate psychiatric/emergency department evaluation if patient is danger to herself, infant, or others
- Headache: need to evaluate blood pressure (rule out preeclampsia), possible epidural headache (postural symptoms)

---

■ Pelvic examination: external genitalia, urethra (lesions, prolapse), bladder (cystocele), vaginal mucosa (discharge, lesions, atrophic), cervix (lesions, friability, color, discharge), uterus (tender, enlarged, position), adnexa (tenderness, masses, fullness), rectum/anus (hemorrhoids, masses, Hemo-occult, rectocele), inguinal lymph nodes

■ Abdominal pain: differential diagnosis in the nonpregnant female includes postovulatory bleeding, ovarian torsion, infections (e.g., STD, PID, UTI), appendicitis, diverticulitis, enlarged ovarian cysts, endometriosis/adenomyosis (see Abdominal Pain)

 **Laboratory Studies**

- Pap smear
- KOH/wet prep/nitrazine if indicated
- Possible cultures, HIV/RPR/hepatitis B and C

 **Pearls**

- Pap smear: adequate Pap needs plus endocervical cells

---

## Amenorrhea

The classic definition of amenorrhea is no period by age 14 and the absence of growth or development of secondary sexual characteristics, or no period by age 16 regardless of normal growth and development and presence of secondary sexual characteristics. Causes of primary amenorrhea include gonadal failure, androgen insensitivity, müllerian duct abnormality, and developmental delay. Causes of secondary amenorrhea include thyroid disease, polycystic ovarian syndrome, premature menopause, pituitary disease, hyperprolactinemia, weight fluctuations (anorexia, athletes, obesity), and Asherman syndrome.

### Pertinent Positives/Negatives

- First day of LMP, childhood growth and development, family history of age of menarche/menopause, duration and flow of menses, cycle days, sexual history
- Exercise history, substance abuse, breast discharge, virilization changes, vasomotor changes, hearing loss, headaches, recent weight loss/gain

##  Physical Examination

■ Measure height/weight

■ Assess sexual development (breast growth, axillary/pubic hair, genitalia), galactorrhea, signs of virilization

## Laboratory Studies

■ β-hCG, prolactin

■ CBC, TSH, bone age, FSH/LH, progestin challenge, total testosterone, DHEA-S

## Pearls

■ Rule out pregnancy in all patients with amenorrhea.

---

## Abnormal/Dysfunctional Uterine Bleeding

Menstrual bleeding is considered abnormal if it occurs more frequently than every 3 weeks or if the flow lasts longer than 7–8 days. Pregnancy, miscarriage/abortion, uterine fibroids, endometrial polyps, endometritis, endometrial hyperplasia, endometriosis, foreign body, and cervical and endometrial cancer should be considered.

■ Menorrhagia: excessive or prolonged menses

■ Metrorrhagia: irregular menses

■ Menometrorrhagia: irregular, prolonged, heavy menstrual bleeding

### Pertinent Positives/Negatives

■ First day of LMP, amount of menstruation now vs. normal cycle, number of pads per day, abdominal pain, length of time patient has had irregular periods, sexual activity, trauma, time of last pelvic examination, contraceptive use, previous miscarriages

- Orthostatic symptoms, recent weight loss/gain, increased fatigue, history of anemia, anticoagulant use
- Use of over-the-counter medications, hormone supplements

## Physical Examination

- Orthostatic BP, pallor
- Vaginal foreign body, bleeding from os (color: bright red blood versus maroon/dark), palpable uterus with/without masses, adnexal masses, bleeding diathesis, hirsute, palpable ovaries
- Obesity, thyroid findings (thyromegaly, goiter, thyroid nodules)

## Laboratory Studies

- β-hCG, CBC, PT/PTT, TSH, prolactin, FSH, LH, total testosterone
- U/S, Pap smear
- Consider endometrial biopsy

## Management

- Treat the underlying cause
- Correct hypovolemia
- Hormone replacement or oral contraceptive therapy
- D&C in women older than 35 years of age; consider D&C if bleeding is uncontrollable or surgical intervention (uterine artery ligation, hysterectomy, endometrial ablation) if it is unresolved.

## Pearls

- Some clinicians use a cutoff of 24 pads a day for heavy bleeding. (The average pad holds 10–15 mL of blood, and the average tampon holds 5 mL of blood.)

▪ Any postmenopausal woman with dysfunctional uterine bleeding requires an endometrial biopsy to rule out endometrial cancer.

## Lower Genital Tract Infections/Vulvovaginitis

Normal vaginal discharge is white and odorless, with a pH of 4. Patients may be asymptomatic or present with increased vaginal discharge, burning, discomfort, or odor.

### Pertinent Positives/Negatives
▪ Vaginal odor, vaginal discharge, vaginal itching/burning, dyspareunia, vulvar erythema, vaginal bleeding
▪ Abdominal pain, sexual activity/contraception, first day of LMP, urinary symptoms, history of STDs, tight clothing, recent antibiotic use

### Physical Examination
▪ Fever, abdominal tenderness, rebound tenderness
▪ Vaginal discharge, vaginal mucosa, vulvar erythema/ excoriations, external lesions, cervical punctuate hemorrhages, tender adnexa/CMT

### Laboratory Studies
▪ Consider β-hCG, wet "prep," GC/chlamydia, Accu-Chek, UA, nitrazine

### Management
▪ Treat underlying disease
▪ Bacterial vaginosis: *Gardnerella vaginalis* infection; treatment with metronidazole PO/vaginal, clindamycin

- Can be asymptomatic
- Wet "prep": clue cells
- Nitrazine test: turns blue
- Whiff test
- Trichomoniasis (sexually transmitted): *Trichomonas vaginalis* infection; treatment with metronidazole (two-gram one-time dose)
  - Green foamy discharge (usually copious)
  - Males asymptomatic
  - Wet "prep": motile trichomonads
- Candidiasis: *Candida albicans* infection; treatment with antifungals
  - White "cottage cheese" discharge
  - Vaginal/vulvar burning/pruritus
  - Pseudohyphae on KOH stain

## Pearls

- Normal physiologic discharge can pool in the posterior fornix.
- Patients may be embarrassed by vaginal discharge and not offer information; ask if there is discharge on their underwear.
- Patients taking metronidazole should not drink ethyl alcohol due to disulfiram-like reaction.
- In recurrent candidal infections (or patients with no medical follow-up), consider HIV or DM.

## Upper Genital Tract Infections/Pelvic Inflammatory Disease (PID)

PID and related infections are characterized by polymicrobial infection/inflammation of the upper genital tract.

The incidence of this condition is increasing in the United States. Patients present with abdominal pain, discharge, and bleeding, or they may be asymptomatic. Complications include tubo-ovarian abscess, infertility, and chronic pain.

## Pertinent Positives/Negatives

■ Fever, abdominal and/or pelvic pain, vaginal discharge, bleeding, nausea/vomiting, anorexia, onset/type of pain, sexual activity/contraception, multiple sexual partners, urinary symptoms, low back pain

■ Use of IUDs, history of endometriosis, history of STDs, first day of LMP, previous surgeries

## Physical Examination

■ Fever, abdominal tenderness/guarding/rebound/peritoneal signs

■ CMT, uterine/adnexal tenderness, cervical discharge, RUQ pain (Fitz-Hugh-Curtis syndrome)

■ Jaundice, CVA tenderness, rectal tenderness, decreased bowel sounds, surgical scars

## Laboratory Studies

■ β-hCG, CBC, ESR, CRP, wet "prep"/GC/chlamydia, UA

■ Consider U/S, RPR, HIV testing, culdocentesis

## Management

■ Antibiotics, correct hypovolemia

■ Consider admission, possible surgery for tubo-ovarian abscess

## Pearls

■ Clinical criteria for diagnosis of PID: abdominal tenderness, CMT, adnexal tenderness, ± fever, leukocytosis, purulent fluid on laparoscopy/culdocentesis, pelvic abscess

- "Chandelier" sign: severe CMT on examination
- *Neisseria gonorrhoeae* and *Chlamydia trachomatis*: traditionally considered the most common pathogens

---

## Sexually Transmitted Disease (STD)

STD is infection of the lower genital tract/external genitalia. It is one of the most common infections in the United States. More than 20 types isolated. Genital herpes is the most common STD in women. Infection with some STDs increase the likelihood of infection with HIV infection or hepatitis B.

### Pertinent Positives/Negatives
- Fever, discharge, dysuria, dyspareunia, postcoital bleeding, pelvic discomfort
- Abdominal pain, nausea, vomiting, anorexia, skin rash, pruritus, jaundice, night sweats, arthralgias/arthritis
- Urinary symptoms, genital lesions/chancres, viral syndrome, weight loss
- History of STD, sexual history, recent international travel, use of contraception, multiple sexual partners, previous HIV testing/blood donation

### Physical Examination
- Fever, abdominal pain
- CMT, uterine/adnexal tenderness, cervical/vaginal discharge, rash, skin lesions, vaginal/rectal skin lesions
- Joint swelling, cachexia, lymphadenopathy

## 🔬 Laboratory Studies

- β-hCG, CBC, ESR/CRP, wet prep/GC/chlamydia, UA, RPR/FTA-ABS, hepatitis profile
- Consider skin biopsy, HIV testing

## 💊 Management

- Treat underlying disorder
- Educate patient about STD prevention; emphasize contraception, informing partner, and medication compliance
- Consider HIV testing
- Inquire about drug use

## ✴ Pearls

- HIV screening tests may not be positive for 3–6 months after inoculation. Females are more likely to be asymptomatic. Some states require counseling when HIV testing is performed.
- Prolonged STD infection may lead to infertility, increased risk of ectopic pregnancy, chronic pelvic pain, and malignancy (especially cervical cancer from HPV).

# 7 Renal/Genitourinary System

## Evaluation of Hematuria

Hematuria is a common complaint; the incidence of painless hematuria is 3%–4%. Generally, hematuria is defined as greater than 5 RBC/hpf. As little as 1 mL of blood in 1 L can cause appreciable hematuria. There are multiple causes of hematuria, both renal and nonrenal. The most common causes are kidney stones, carcinoma of the kidney or bladder, urethritis, UTIs, BPH, and glomerulonephritis. Table 7-1 presents the differential diagnosis of hematuria.

### Pertinent Positives/Negatives: OPQRST

- **O**nset: when and how symptoms began
- **P**rovocative/**P**alliative: not applicable
- **Q**uality: painful or painless hematuria; associated with abdominal, back, or flank pain; bleeding disorders, recent infection
- **R**egion/**R**adiation: blood noticed only at initiation of voiding, continuously, or with the last few drops of urine; occurrence of clots; frequency and quality of hematuria (red, pink, brown, smoky colored urine)
- **S**everity: 1 to 10
- **T**iming: constant or intermittent

Associated features: fever or chills, dysuria, nocturia, vaginal bleeding, pregnancy, abdominal mass, prostatic disease, history of kidney disease (family history), bleeding disorders,

### TABLE 7-1
## Differential Diagnosis of Hematuria

Renal causes: papillary necrosis, renal artery embolism, proliferative nephritides, membranoproliferative, lupus nephritis, IgA nephropathy (Berger disease), postexercise, severe hypertension, lymphoma, amyloidosis, polycystic renal disease, paroxysmal nocturnal hematuria

Other: kidney stones, neoplasms, BPH, infections (UTI), menstruation, urethral trauma, vaginal lacerations/bleeding, rectal bleeding, urethral strictures, endometriosis, AAA, myoglobinuria, drugs (phenazopyridine, rifampin)

sore throat, tobacco use, medications, recent treatment for UTI, atrial fibrillation, sickle cell disease, strenuous exercise, TB exposure

 **Physical Examination**

■ Fever, tachycardia or bradycardia, hypertension or hypotension, orthostatic vital signs, AMS, CVA tenderness, abdominal pain, palpable masses, hepatosplenomegaly, arthritis, irregular heart beat, cutaneous evidence of bleeding

■ Urethral lesions

■ Rectal examination with prostate examination, pelvic examination

 **Laboratory Studies (Table 7-2)**

■ CBC, CMP, UA (with microscopic examination)

■ Consider AAS, CT, U/S, biopsy

 **Management**

■ Treat underlying disorder

■ Correct hypovolemia

---

**TABLE 7-2**

## Criteria for Diagnostic Work-Up of Hematuria

1. Suspicion of malignancy

2. Two of three urinalyses showing 3 or more RBCs/hpf

3. One urinalysis showing more than 100 RBCs/hpf

4. Any single episode of gross hematuria and both of the following:

   a. No clear reason for benign, transient, hematuria (e.g., vigorous exercise, minor trauma, bladder catheterization, sexual activity) **and**

   b. No obvious diagnostic clue (e.g., dysuria or pyuria suggesting UTI)

(From Frances C, Bent S, and Saint S. (eds.) Saint-Frances Guide to Outpatient Medicine. Philadelphia: Lippincott Williams & Wilkins, 2002:258.)

❀ **Pearls**

▪ RBCs in the urine with a history typical of nephrolithiasis in the elderly is AAA until proven otherwise.

---

## Evaluation of Renal Failure

Renal failure can be classified as acute or chronic. This discussion will be limited to ARF, which is a sudden decrease in kidney function resulting in a rapid increase in the retention of BUN and Cr. There may or may not be a change in urine output. ARF can be classified as prerenal, intrinsic, or postrenal. ARF is often transient and reversible. Prerenal causes include hypovolemia, sepsis, shock, drugs, renal artery stenosis, and decreased cardiac output. Intrinsic causes include acute tubular necrosis, glomerulonephritis, nephritis, and acute interstitial nephritis. Postrenal causes include nephrolithiasis, prostate disease, bladder neck obstruction (cancer), and urethral strictures.

## Pertinent Positives/Negatives: OPQRST

■ **O**nset: when and how symptoms began

■ **P**rovocative/**P**alliative: not applicable

■ **Q**uality: back, abdominal, flank, or groin pain; chest pain and/or dyspnea

■ **R**egion/**R**adiation: not applicable

■ **S**everity: 1 to 10

■ **T**iming: constant or intermittent symptoms

Associated with previous history of kidney disease (Table 7-3)

 **Physical Examination**

■ Fever, tachycardia or bradycardia, hypotension or hypertension, orthostatic vital signs, skin turgor (hydration status), AMS, pericardial friction rub, JVD, evidence of peripheral edema, CVA tenderness, presence of mediport, asterixis, jaundice

■ Urine output (check)

■ Abdominal examination (feel for outlet obstruction)

### TABLE 7-3
### Conditions Previously Associated with Acute Renal Failure

• Prerenal: bleeding, trauma or burns, vomiting or diarrhea, dehydration, evidence of CHF, dizziness, weakness, fever, infection, medications (ACE inhibitors, NSAIDs)

• Intrinsic: recent radiographic imaging with dye, medications, previous infection, hematuria, cough

• Postrenal: back/flank pain, difficulty urinating, self-catheterization, dysuria, weight loss, history of prostate problems, recent instrumentation

### Laboratory Studies
- CBC, CMP (especially BUN/Cr), UA, urine Cr, urine Na
- Consider AAS, U/S, CT

### Management
- Treat underlying cause; balance fluids and electrolytes
  - Prerenal: volume replacement/management
  - Intrinsic: discontinue offending agents, increase kidney perfusion/output (hydration, diuretics, dopamine)
  - Postrenal: catheterization, hydration
- Consider dialysis

### Pearls
- Calculate the fractional excretion of Na ($Fe_{Na}$) to evaluate for prerenal failure:

$$(Urine_{Na}/Plasma_{Na})/(Urine_{Cr}/Plasma_{Cr}) \times 100$$

  If this value is < 1%, then the patient is in prerenal ARF.
- If the patient is on dialysis, ask them their schedule, last visit, and dry weight.
- Differential diagnosis:
  - Prerenal: hypovolemia, CHF, liver failure, sepsis, renal artery stenosis, embolic disease
  - Intrinsic: acute tubular necrosis, ischemia, toxins, autoimmune diseases, acute glomerulonephritis, drug reactions, acute interstitial nephritis
  - Postrenal: urethral obstruction, tubular obstruction from crystals, papillary necrosis, urolithiasis, retroperitoneal tumor

## Nephrolithiasis

Nephrolithiasis, or kidney stones (also with ureteral/cystic stones), is a common condition that usually occurs in the third to fifth decade of life. Both genetic (hypercalciuria, gout, cystinuria) and environmental (hot environment, dehydration, outside workers, medications) factors predispose patients to kidney stones. Urologic stone disease results from a supersaturation of urine with urinary solutes. Crystals precipitate out into the urine and coalesce to form stones (calculi) in the kidney and ureters. Symptoms arise as these calculi obstruct in the renal pelvis or ureters. Classically, patients present with sudden onset of flank pain, associated with nausea, vomiting, "pain worse than childbirth," hematuria, and radiation to the front lower quadrants or groin.

### Pertinent Positives/Negatives: OPQRST

▪ **O**nset: when and how symptoms began, possible history of symptoms or kidney stones

▪ **P**rovocative/**P**alliative: worsens with activity, outside work, dehydration, movement, summertime, alcohol intake; improves with anti-inflammatory medications, hydration

▪ **Q**uality: sudden, sharp onset of flank "colicky" pain; deep, sharp, knife-like pain

▪ **R**egion/**R**adiation: pain starts in flank, radiates anteroinferiorly to abdomen into groin/inner thigh

▪ **S**everity: almost always severe

▪ **T**iming: constant or intermittent

Associated features: nausea, vomiting, diaphoresis, colicky pain ("writhing of renal colic"), anxiety, pacing, inability to lie still, hematuria, frequency, nocturia, back pain, urinary retention (large bladder stone)

## Physical Examination

■ Fever, tachycardia, hypertension, "writhing in pain," unable to lie still, decreased bowel sounds, evidence of dehydration (dry mucosa, no axillary sweat, skin tenting)

■ CVA tenderness, evidence of pulsatile mass in abdomen, normal distal pulses, peritoneal findings (should be negative), no rash

■ Normal testicular examination

## Laboratory Studies

■ CBC, CMP, UA (with hematuria)

■ Consider IVP, CT scan, U/S of kidneys (suspect hydronephrosis, obstruction)

## Management

■ IV fluids, pain medications (NSAIDs or opiates), antiemetic medications, urine strainer

■ If evidence of infection, admission, IV antibiotics, immediate drainage via percutaneous drain or ureteral stent

## Pearls

■ Up to 20% of kidney stones may show no hematuria. The degree of hematuria is not predictive of stone size or likelihood of passage.

■ A urine pH greater than 7.0 suggests presence of urea-splitting organisms, such as *Proteus*.

■ Lloyd's kidney punch sign: pain to deep percussion of kidney

■ RBCs in the urine with a history typical of nephrolithiasis in the elderly is AAA until proven otherwise.

■ CT has a sensitivity or nearly 100% in multiple studies in detecting the presence of stones.

## Pyelonephritis

Pyelonephritis, a condition of bacterial invasion of the renal parenchyma, presents in a patient with symptoms of UTI for several days (dysuria and fever), followed by more systemic symptoms, chills, fever, flank pain, nausea, and vomiting. Illness severity may range from mild infection with few systemic symptoms to ARDS to multiorgan system failure. Factors associated with increased risk of pyelonephritis include pregnancy, prolonged symptoms of UTI before seeking care, recurrent UTIs, chronic urinary catheters, and immunocompromised status (HIV, transplantation, DM). The typical pathogens that cause pyelonephritis are *Escherichia coli* and other coliform bacteria.

### Pertinent Positives/Negatives: OPQRST

■ **O**nset: length of time patient has had urinary frequency/dysuria/nocturia, frequency of past UTIs, length of time catheter has been in place
■ **P**rovocative/**P**alliative: not applicable
■ **Q**uality:  flank pain (dull, ache), fevers, shaking chills
■ **R**egion/**R**adiation: abdominal pain
■ **S**everity: 1 to 10
■ **T**iming: constant or intermittent symptoms

Associated features: fever, chills, nausea, vomiting, dehydration, urinary frequency/dysuria/hesitancy, hematuria, abdominal/suprapubic pain, malaise, weakness, anorexia, possible recent antibiotic use

##  Physical Examination

- Fever, tachycardia, hypotension or hypertension
- Discomfort, CVA tenderness, suprapubic tenderness, evidence of urologic instrumentation, lack of peritoneal signs
- Normal pelvic examination

## Laboratory Studies

- CBC, CMP, pregnancy test, UA, urine culture, blood culture
- Consider CT/US

## Management (Table 7-4)

- IV fluids, antipyretics, antibiotics (typically fluoroquinolones)

---

## Testicular Pain

---

Many conditions can refer pain to the testicles, including life-threatening disorders such as Fournier gangrene (scrotal necrotizing fasciitis) and a ruptured aortic aneurysm. Many limb-threatening conditions (testicular torsion, paraphimosis) should also quickly be evaluated. Often the patient is extremely nervous and may give a limited history due to embarrassment or baseline mental status (the elderly or alcoholics).

### Pertinent Positive/Negatives: OPQRST

- **O**nset: when and how symptoms began, history of symptoms, patient's activity when symptoms began (what was he doing when he noticed symptoms?)

**TABLE 7-4**

Treatment of Urinary Tract Infections

| Type of Infection | Microorganisms | Treatment | Disposition |
|---|---|---|---|
| Uncomplicated cystitis | • *Escherichia coli*<br>• *Staphylococcus saprophyticus*<br>• *Proteus mirabilis*<br>• *Klebsiella pneumoniae* | • 3 days<br>• Trimethoprim-sulfamethoxazole<br>• Ciprofloxacin<br>• Norfloxacin<br>• Ofloxacin<br>• Amoxicillin-clavulanate<br>• Levofloxacin | • Home |
| Uncomplicated pyelonephritis | • *Escherichia coli*<br>• *Staphylococcus saprophyticus*<br>• *Proteus mirabilis*<br>• *Klebsiella pneumoniae* | • 10–14 days<br>• Ceftriaxone<br>• Ampicillin plus gentamicin<br>• Levofloxacin<br>• Ciprofloxacin<br>• Amoxicillin-clavulanate | • First dose of IV antibiotics in emergency department<br>• If young and healthy, discharge home with oral antibiotics |

*(Continued)*

149

## TABLE 7-4

### Treatment of Urinary Tract Infections (*continued*)

| Type of Infection | Microorganisms | Treatment | Disposition |
|---|---|---|---|
| Uncomplicated cystitis in pregnancy | • *Escherichia coli*<br>• *Staphylococcus saprophyticus*<br>• *Proteus mirabilis*<br>• *Klebsiella pneumoniae* | • 7–10 days<br>• Amoxicillin<br>• Nitrofurantoin | • Home |
| Complicated urinary tract infection | • *Escherichia coli*<br>• *Staphylococcus saprophyticus*<br>• *Proteus mirabilis*<br>• *Klebsiella pneumoniae*<br>• *Enterobacter* spp.<br>• *Pseudomonas aeruginosa*<br>• Group D streptococci<br>• *Serratia*<br>• *Morganella*<br>• *Staphylococcus aureus*<br>• *Candida* species | • IV antibiotic<br>• Ciprofloxacin<br>• Levofloxacin<br>• Ampicillin plus gentamicin<br>• Cefotaxime<br>• Ceftriaxone<br>• Ticarcillin-clavulanate | • Admission |

(*From Mick N, et al. Blueprints Emergency Medicine, 2nd ed.: Blackwell Publishing, 2006:154.*)

■ **P**rovocative/**P**alliative: worsens with strenuous activity, movement, sexual activity, athletic event, or trauma before onset of pain; improves with lifting scrotum, changing position

■ **Q**uality: sudden sharp pain; swelling or discoloration to penis

■ **R**egion/**R**adiation: pain radiates to groin, scrotum, or inner thigh

■ **S**everity: 1 to 10

■ **T**iming: constant or intermittent

Associated features: nausea, vomiting, fever, rash, dysuria, urinary frequency, penile discharge, swelling, sexual activity, homosexual, age (< 40 years of age = STD, > 40 years of age = urinary pathogens)

 **Physical Examination**

■ Fever, tachycardia, hypotension or hypertension

■ Inability to lie still, swollen testis, firm/tender scrotum (often higher in the scrotum on torsion, horizontal lie), inability to retract foreskin easily, penile discharge, normal pulses, discoloration/gangrenous changes to scrotal wall

 **Laboratory Studies**

■ CBC, CMP, UA

■ Consider testicular ultrasound/CT

 **Management**

■ Case specific

■ Testicular torsion = detorsion

■ Phimosis (inability to retract the foreskin proximally) = circumcision/steroids

- Paraphimosis (inability to reduce the proximal foreskin distally) = compression of glans/detumescence
- Fournier gangrene (polymicrobial necrotizing fasciitis of perineal fascia) = antibiotics, fluid resuscitation, surgical debridement
- AAA = surgery

## ✿ Pearls

- Fournier gangrene is most common in males with diabetes (females can develop perineal fasciitis as well).
- Prehn sign = relief of pain with elevation of affected testicle (cannot reliably distinguish torsion from epididymitis)

# 8 Metabolic System

## DIABETES

### Diabetes Mellitus Type 1

Type 1 DM, also known as juvenile-onset IDDM, is characterized by the inability of the pancreas to secrete insulin, possibly secondary to autoimmune destruction of the beta cells of the pancreas. Patients initially diagnosed with IDDM are usually young and lean and present with DKA secondary to the lack of insulin.

#### Pertinent Positives/Negatives: OPQRST

- **O**nset: type of diabetes the patient has, length of time the patient has had diabetes, how does the patient administer insulin to self (pump vs. subcutaneous)
- **P**rovocative/**P**alliative: frequency with which patient checks his or her blood glucose; time of patient's last HgbA$_{1C}$; hypoglycemic episodes, if any; time of patient's last eye examination; frequent, problematic infections, if any
- **Q**uality: not applicable
- **R**egion/**R**adiation: any symptoms of uncontrolled diabetes, whether short term (polyuria, polydipsia) or long term (vision loss, neuropathy, nephropathy, poor healing wounds)?
- **S**everity: difficulty of control of diabetes
- **T**iming: not applicable

Miscellaneous: polyphagia, nocturia, fatigue, weight loss (unintentional), frequent infections (candidiasis, balanitis), family history of DM, AMS, medications (steroids), recent infection or stress, abdominal pain, nausea/vomiting, weakness

## Physical Examination

■ Fever, hypotension or hypertension, tachycardia or bradycardia, orthostatic symptoms/vital signs
■ AMS, skin turgor, mucous membranes, evidence of infection, acetone (fruity) odor
■ Foot examination for foreign bodies/ulcers
■ Eye examination for retinopathy

## Laboratory Studies

■ Accu-Chek, CBC, CMP, UA, serum/urine ketones
■ Consider ECG

## Management

■ Treat for DKA if present
■ Correct hypovolemia/electrolyte abnormalities
■ Insulin

## Pearls

■ Necrobiosis lipoidica is a well-demarcated, red, atrophic rash that usually appears on the anterior shin of diabetic patients. Its cause is unknown.
■ Be sure to ask the patient the type and amount of insulin they use, as well as the time given (Table 8-1).

| TABLE 8-1 |
| --- |

## Insulin Pharmacokinetics

| Insulin | Preparation | Onset (h) | Peak (h) | Duration (h) |
| --- | --- | --- | --- | --- |
| Rapid acting | Regular | 0.5–1.0 | 2.5–5.0 | 8–12 |
| | Lispro (Humalog) | 0.25 | 0.5–1.5 | 2–5 |
| | Aspart (NovoLog) | 0.25 | 1–3 | 3–5 |
| Intermediate acting | NPH | 1.0–1.5 | 4–12 | 24 |
| | Lente | 1.0–2.5 | 7–15 | 24 |
| Long acting | Glargine (Lantus) | Throughout 24-hour period (no peak) | | |
| | Ultralente | 2–8 | 10–30 | 20–36 |

## Diabetes Mellitus Type 2

Type 2 DM, also known as adult-onset NIDDM, is characterized by hyperglycemia secondary to peripheral insulin resistance and decreased insulin secretion. It generally occurs in
obese people older than 40 years of age, and patients have
a strong family history of NIDDM. Patients undiagnosed with
NIDDM may present with polyuria, polydipsia, or polyphagia, but often the diagnosis is made incidentally on routine
laboratory studies. Patients with NIDDM present in a nonketotic hyperosmolar state, unlike patients with IDDM, who
present with DKA.

### Pertinent Positives/Negatives: OPQRST

■ **O**nset: type of diabetes the patient has, length of time
the patient has had diabetes, how patient treats his or her

diabetes (diet, exercise, medication; medication in combination with insulin)

■ **P**rovocative/**P**alliative: frequency with which patient checks his or her blood glucose; time of patient's last HgbA$_{1C}$; hypoglycemic episodes, if any; time of patient's last eye examination; frequent, problematic infections, if any

■ **Q**uality: not applicable

■ **R**egion/**R**adiation: any symptoms of uncontrolled diabetes, whether short term (polyuria, polydipsia) or long term (vision loss, neuropathy, nephropathy, poor healing wounds)

■ **S**everity: difficulty of control of diabetes

■ **T**iming: not applicable

Miscellaneous: polyuria, polydipsia, polyphagia, nocturia, fatigue, weight loss (unintentional), frequent infections (candidiasis, balanitis), family history of DM, AMS, medications (steroids), recent infection/stress, abdominal pain, nausea/vomiting, blurry vision, weakness, paresthesias/numbness, erectile dysfunction

### Physical Examination

■ Fever, hypotension or hypertension, tachycardia or bradycardia, orthostatic vital signs

■ AMS, skin turgor, mucous membranes, evidence of infection, acetone (fruity) odor, evidence of neuropathy, peripheral pulse examination "stocking glove distribution," lower extremity hyperpigmentation, necrobiosis lipoidica diabeticorum

### Laboratory Studies

■ Accu-Chek, CBC, CMP, UA, serum/urine ketones, HgbA$_{1c}$

■ Consider ECG, cardiac enzymes

### 💊 Management

■ Treat for nonketotic hyperosmolar state if present

■ Oral hypoglycemics and other medications

■ Treat for concomitant infections and electrolyte abnormalities

## Diabetic Ketoacidosis (DKA)

DKA is a hyperglycemia-induced emergency that occurs more commonly in IDDM but can also occur in NIDDM. The lack of insulin production causes hyperglycemia, resulting in an osmotic diuresis, followed by severe dehydration and electrolyte disturbances (especially potassium). The formation of ketones from fatty acid oxidation occurs because muscle and fat are not able to take up glucose. Acidosis results from ketone depletion of acid buffers cellularly and extracellularly. The most common causes of DKA are infection, noncompliance, and stressors (MI, stroke, pregnancy), as well as undiagnosed IDDM.

### Pertinent Positives/Negatives: OPQRST

■ **O**nset: length of time the patient has been feeling weak/sick, length of time the patient has had diabetes, how the patient controls his or her diabetes, whether the patient ran out of diabetic medication, time that the patient last checked his or her blood glucose

■ **P**rovocative/**P**alliative: not applicable

■ **Q**uality: not applicable

■ **R**egion/**R**adiation: possible chest pain, weakness, abdominal pain, or fever

- **S**everity: not applicable
- **T**iming: possible history of hospital admission for high blood sugar

Miscellaneous: type and severity of DM, medication compliance, AMS/confusion, fevers/chills, chest pain/discomfort/dyspnea, evidence of any infection (especially urinary), productive cough, polyuria, polydipsia, nocturia, thirst, nausea/vomiting, lethargy, weakness, dizziness, anorexia/increased appetite, abdominal pain, recent trauma, weakness, slurred speech

### Factors That Precipitate DKA: 5 Is

**I**nfection
**I**schemia (cardiac, mesenteric)
**I**nfarction
**I**gnorance (poor control)
**I**ntoxication (alcohol)

## Physical Examination

- Fever, tachycardia or bradycardia, hypotension, tachypnea, orthostatic symptoms/vital signs
- AMS, dry mucous membranes, poor skin turgor, no perspiration, oral candidiasis, acetone/fruity breath, abdominal tenderness, back pain, vaginal discharge, rhonchi/rales, recent surgical scars, neurologic deficits

## Laboratory Studies

- Accu-Chek (high), CBC, CMP, UA, serum/urine ketones, cardiac enzymes, ECG, CXR
- Consider AAS, ABG

## 🔖 Management

■ Aggressive fluid administration (patients can be deficient of up to 10 L)

■ Insulin, potassium replacement with rehydration

■ Manage precipitating factor of DKA

## ❎ Pearls

■ Abdominal pain in DKA is directly proportional to serum ketone levels.

■ DKA is associated with anion gap metabolic acidosis.

■ Hypokalemia can be life-threatening once treatment for DKA has been initiated; consider replacing potassium.

■ Bicarbonate should rarely be used in the treatment of DKA (it can worsen intracellular acidosis).

## Electrolyte Disturbances

### Hypercalcemia

Hypercalcemia is defined as a serum calcium >10.5 mg/dL or an ionized calcium of >2.7 mEq/L. Severe hypercalcemia, or hypercalcemic crisis, is the presence of acute symptoms and a serum level >14 mg/dL. Hypercalcemia has several causes, but malignancy and hyperparathyroidism are the two most common and must be ruled out.

### Causes

■ Malignancy (especially lung, myeloma, leukemia, breast, kidney), hyperparathyroidism

- Paget disease, calcium supplementation, vitamin A or D intoxication, adrenal insufficiency, medications (lithium and thiazides especially), sarcoidosis, immobilization

### Hypercalcemia: MD PIMPS ME

**M**alignancy
**D**iuretics (thiazide the main culprit)
**P**arathyroid (hyperparathyroidism)
**I**mmobilization/**I**diopathic
**M**egadoses of vitamins A, D
**P**aget disease
**S**arcoidosis
**M**ilk alkali syndrome
**E**ndocrine (Addison disease, thyrotoxicosis)

## Signs and Symptoms

- Initially: asymptomatic
- Irritability, anorexia, nausea, vomiting, confusion, weakness, fatigue, constipation, abdominal pain, weight loss, polyuria, weakness, polydipsia, nephrolithiasis, joint complaints/ bony pain, hypertension, coma

## ECG Findings

- QT shortening, prolonged PR, increased QRS, T wave changes, heart block

###  Management

- IV hydration, furosemide (Lasix) (avoid thiazides, because they increase calcium)
- Treat underlying cause (calcitonin, glucocorticoids).
- Consider calcitonin, diphosphonates, mithramycin, gallium, EDTA, dialysis, plicamycin, or prednisone (for malignancy).

## ❇ Pearls

■ Rhyme: **bones** (bony pain and pathologic fractures), **stones** (kidney stones and polyuria), **groans** (abdominal pain, nausea, vomiting, anorexia, ileus), and psychiatric **moans** (AMS, depression, psychosis)

■ Severe hypercalcemia can cause nephrocalcinosis and renal failure from calcium deposits in the kidney.

■ EDTA at 50 mg/kg IV only in life-threatening features

■ Use calcium-free dialysate in dialysis patients.

■ If furosemide is used, urine output should be kept at 200–300 mL/hr.

## Hypocalcemia

Hypocalcemia is defined as a serum calcium < 8.5 mg/dL or an ionized calcium < 2.0 mEq/L and is more common than hypercalcemia. Morbidity for hypocalcemia itself is much less than hypercalcemia. The causes of hypocalcemia, however, carry a great morbidity. The classic sign of hypocalcemia is tetany.

### Causes

■ Hypoalbuminemia (cirrhosis, nephrosis, sepsis, chronic illness, burns), alkalosis (effects on ionized fraction of calcium), pancreatitis, drugs (cimetidine, aminoglycosides, loop diuretics), hypoparathyroidism (postsurgery or intrinsic), malnutrition, renal failure (vitamin D metabolism), vitamin D deficiency, tumorlysis syndrome

### Signs and Symptoms

■ Tetany

■ Cramping, weakness, fatigue, dyspnea, hand/feet paresthesias, perioral paresthesias, distal numbness, vomiting, hyperactive reflexes, hypotension, seizures, CHF

## ECG Findings
- Prolonged QT interval

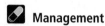 **Management**
- Administer calcium PO/IV, vitamin D.
- Treat underlying cause.

### ❀ Pearls
- Chvostek sign: tapping facial nerve below zygoma induces contraction of facial muscles
- Trousseau sign: inflating BP cuff above systolic BP in upper extremity causes nerve ischemia, resulting in carpal spasm
- Remember that phosphorus and calcium levels are usually in the opposite direction.
- A decrease in serum albumin of 1 g/dL decreases total serum Ca 0.8 mg/dL.
- IV calcium can cause hypotension and tissue necrosis; consider a central line.
- Correct magnesium as well as calcium.

## Hyperkalemia

Increased potassium (>5.0 mEq/L) is a potentially life-threatening condition. Patients may be asymptomatic but may present with weakness, paresthesias, nausea or vomiting, muscle cramps, paralysis, confusion, respiratory insufficiency, or full cardiac arrest. Because hyperkalemia may result in cardiac arrest secondary to arrhythmia, any suggestion of increased potassium should prompt a physician to obtain an immediate ECG and draw a serum potassium.

## Causes

■ Laboratory error: hemolysis, leukocytosis, thrombocytosis, improper blood collection

■ Decreased excretion: acute or chronic renal failure, urinary obstruction, medications (ACE inhibitors, NSAIDs, potassium-sparing diuretics), Addison disease, sickle cell anemia

■ Increased potassium in extracellular space: acidosis, anemia, trauma, chemotherapy, mineralocorticoid deficiency, potassium supplements, rhabdomyolysis, burns, succinylcholine, hemolysis, acute digoxin toxicity, beta-blockers

## Signs and Symptoms

■ Asymptomatic presentation, generalized fatigue, weakness, paresthesias, palpitations, nausea, vomiting, diarrhea, confusion, hypotension, arrhythmias, cardiac arrest

## ECG Findings

■ $K^+$ = 5.0–6.0 mEq/L: peaked T waves

■ $K^+$ = 6.0–7.0 mEq/L: prolonged PR/QT intervals, flat P waves, depressed ST segments

■ $K^+$ = 7.0–8.0 mEq/L: widened QRS

■ $K^+$ = 8.0–10.0 mEq/L: sine wave (ventricular fibrillation/asystole)

## Management

■ Verify hyperkalemia with ECG and repeat serum $K^+$.

■ Calcium gluconate stabilizes the cardiac membrane.

■ Albuterol treatments, insulin and glucose, or sodium bicarbonate temporarily shifts potassium into cells.

■ Furosemide (Lasix) promotes renal excretion of potassium.

- Sodium polystyrene sulfonate (Kayexalate) exchanges potassium for sodium in the gut (takes up to 2 hours).
- Dialysis can be used for severe cases or patients in renal failure.

## Hypokalemia

Decreased potassium (less than 3.5 mEq/L) is often not as life-threatening as hyperkalemia but is considered severe when potassium is less than 2.5 mEq/L. Severe hypokalemia is relatively uncommon. Muscle weakness is the most common symptom.

### Causes
- Alkalosis (hyperventilating)
- Medications: diuretics (especially loop diuretics), insulin, albuterol, bicarbonate, gentamicin, penicillins
- Renal losses: magnesium deficiency, renal tubular acidosis, hyperaldosteronism
- GI losses: diarrhea, vomiting, laxative use, NG tube suctioning, fistulas, decreased intake
- Other conditions: familial hypokalemic periodic paralysis

### Signs and Symptoms
- Weakness, fatigue, cramps, ileus, paresthesias, palpitations, psychosis, depression, dehydration, nephrogenic diabetes insipidus, autonomic instability (hypotension), arrhythmias, areflexia, respiratory failure, AMS

### ECG Findings
- $K^+$ < 3.0 mEq/L: low-voltage QRS, flat T waves, prominent P waves

■ $K^+ < 2.5$ mEq/L: prominent U waves
■ $K^+ < 2.0$ mEq/L: widened QRS

### 🔖 Management

■ Treat the underlying disorder (stop diuretics)
■ Potassium supplementation (PO/IV)
■ Replace magnesium deficiency if present.

### ✳️ Pearls

■ In *al-kay-LOW-sis* (alkalosis), potassium is LOW.
■ Do not replace potassium too quickly (~20 mEq/hr IV or PO).
■ Giving 10 mEq of KCl increases the serum $K^+$ approximately 0.1 mEq.
■ Ensure adequate urine output/renal function before giving potassium.
■ It is difficult, if not impossible, to treat hypokalemia if the patient is magnesium deficient.

## Hypernatremia

Hypernatremia, defined as a serum sodium > 145 mEq/L, is rare in the healthy individual with an intact thirst response who can respond with increased water intake. However, the condition can develop quickly in patients with kidney pathology or loss of central neurohormonal control. Symptoms are similar to hyponatremia, with confusion, fatigue, AMS, cramps, seizures, and coma.

## Causes

- Renal losses: diabetes insipidus (nephrogenic or central), adrenal/kidney disease, diuretics, postobstructive renal diuresis
- GI losses: decreased thirst (especially elderly, behavioral, or those with hypothalamic lesions), vomiting, diarrhea, fistulas (dehydration with poor supplementation)
- Other: hypertonic saline, insensible losses, salt ingestion, medications (lithium)

**Hypernatremia: 6 Ds**

**D**iuretics
**D**ehydration
**D**iabetes insipidus
**D**ocs (iatrogenic)
**D**iarrhea
**D**isease (e.g., kidney, sickle cell)

## Signs and Symptoms

- Irritability, lethargy, anorexia, recent history of fluid loss (vomiting, diarrhea, fistulas), "doughy" skin, AMS, spasticity/twitching, ataxia, areflexia, seizures, coma

## ECG Findings: none

 **Management**

- Determine if hypervolemic (sodium > water), diuretics, and $D_5W$
- Hypovolemic (water deficit > sodium deficit), correct with NS
- Euvolemic (renal losses), hypotonic fluids

## ❄ Pearls

■ Correct hyponatremia slowly (if quickly, brain edema can result).

■ Lower $Na^+$ no faster than 2 mEq/L per hour.

■ Use intranasal DDAVP for central diabetes insipidus.

---

## Hyponatremia

Hyponatremia is defined as a serum sodium less than 135 mEq/L but can be subdivided into three categories based on serum osmolarity: hypotonic (three different subtypes), isotonic, and hypertonic. It is important to measure the serum osmolality, and volume Hyponatremia can be viewed as an "excess water state." Patients may complain of confusion, seizures, AMS, fatigue, cramps, and coma.

### Causes

■ Hypotonic
  ■ Isovolemic: renal failure, SIADH, medications, hypopituitarism
  ■ Hypovolemic: vomiting, diarrhea, burns, renal losses, Addison disease, diuretics
  ■ Hypervolemic: cirrhosis, nephrotic syndrome, CHF
■ Isotonic: isotonic infusions (glucose, mannitol), or pseudo-hyponatremia (increased glucose, lipids, or serum proteins)
■ Hypertonic: hypertonic infusions (glucose)

### Signs and Symptoms

■ Asymptomatic presentation, confusion, AMS, weakness, depressed reflexes, cramps, nausea, lethargy, hypothermia, pseudobulbar palsies

■ Severe hyponatremia: possible seizures, bradycardia, respiratory arrest, coma

## ECG Findings: none

### 💊 Management

■ Severe hyponatremia (CNS manifestations): consider 3% saline, but with slow correction (no more than 1.0 mEq/L per hour).

■ Consider furosemide (Lasix).

### ❄ Pearls

■ Correcting the sodium too quickly can result in central pontine myelinolysis, which may present as "locked-in syndrome."

■ Legionnaires disease can cause hyponatremia.

■ Serum sodium is diluted by a factor of 1.6 mEq/L for each 100 mg/dL increase in serum glucose.

■ In a surgical patient, the most common cause of hyponatremia is excessive fluid administration.

■ 3% NaCl = 513 mEq/L

■ $Na^+$ deficit formula: $kg \times 0.6 \times (desired\ Na^+ - known\ Na^+)$

■ 3% NaCl drip rate (mL/hr) = patient's mass (kg) × (0.6 or 0.5 L/kg) × (1 to 2 mEq/L/hr)

# 9 | Neurology System

## Cerebrovascular Accident (CVA)

CVA, or "stroke," is the acute neurologic deficit caused by the sudden loss of circulation to the brain. CVAs can be classified as either ischemic (80%; thrombotic/embolic) or hemorrhagic (20%; ICHs/SAHs). TIAs are neurological deficits that resolve within 24 hours. It is important to recognize CVAs as early as possible, because the sooner that therapeutic measures can be instituted, the better the patient outcome.

### Stroke Risk Factors: HEADS

**H**ypertension/**H**yperlipidemia
**E**lderly
**A**trial fibrillation
**D**iabetes mellitus/**D**rugs (cocaine)
**S**moking/**S**ex (male)

## Pertinent Positives/Negatives: OPQRST

- **O**nset: when and how symptoms began (environment, activity on symptoms starting, witnesses), exact time of onset of symptoms
- **P**rovocative/**P**alliative: any history of similar episodes
- **Q**uality: specific neurologic deficit (aphasia, paresis, visual changes or deficits, dysarthria, ataxia, vertigo, AMS)
- **R**egion/**R**adiation: seizures, nausea or vomiting, headache
- **S**everity: 1 to 10
- **T**iming: constant or intermittent

Associated features: trauma; dizziness or weakness; previous CVA, TIA, or CAD; AF; fever; heart murmur; valve replacement; cardiomyopathy; DM; hypertension; hypercholesterolemia; sickle cell anemia; history of blood clots; medications (especially warfarin, ASA, heparin, clopidogrel); recent surgery; history of cancer (intracranial vs. other)

##  Physical Examination

- Fever, hypertension, bradycardia or tachycardia
- Mental status examination, GCS (Table 9-1), detailed neurologic examination (speech, ocular movement, pupils, visual fields, cranial nerve examination, motor/sensory, cerebellar examination, gait, deep tendon reflexes; Table 9-2)
- Signs of trauma, nuchal rigidity, irregular pulse, murmurs, peripheral pulses, carotid bruits, contractures

## Laboratory Studies

- Immediate CT scan (to rule out hemorrhagic CVA), CBC, CMP, Accu-Chek, PT/PT/INR, cardiac enzymes
- Consider UA, UDS, BAL, echocardiography, carotid U/S

## Pearls

- A GCS of 8 should prompt one to consider securing an airway (see Table 9-1).
- Middle cerebral artery distribution: aphasia or neglect, gaze preference
- Anterior communicating artery distribution: contralateral lower extremity paresis, personality changes, AMS
- Posterior cerebral artery distribution: homonymous hemianopsia, AMS, visual disturbances

### TABLE 9-1

## Glasgow Coma Score

**Best Eye Response (4)**

1   No eye opening
2   Eye opening to pain
3   Eye opening to verbal command
4   Eyes open spontaneously

**Best Verbal Response (5)**

1   No verbal response
2   Incomprehensible sounds
3   Inappropriate words
4   Confused
5   Orientated

**Best Motor Response (6)**

1   No motor response
2   Extension to pain
3   Flexion to pain
4   Withdrawal from pain
5   Localizing pain
6   Obeys command

Note: The GCS is scored between 3 and 15, 3 being the worst and 15 the best. It is composed of three parameters: Best Eye Response, Best Verbal Response, and Best Motor Response. A score of 13 or higher correlates with a mild brain injury, 9 to 12 a moderate brain injury, and 8 or less a severe brain injury.

■ Vertebrobasilar distribution: cranial nerve deficits, vertigo, nystagmus, diplopia, dysphagia, coma
■ Lacunar distribution: motor or sensory deficit
■ Wernicke aphasia: fluent, expressive, wordy speech (makes no sense)
■ Broca aphasia: nonfluent, short, "broken" speech

### TABLE 9-2

## National Institutes of Health Stroke Scale for the Assessment of Neurologic Disability

### 1.a. Level of consciousness

| | |
|---|---|
| 0 | Alert |
| 1 | Not alert, but arousable with minimal stimulation |
| 2 | Not alert, requires repeated stimulation to attend |
| 3 | Coma |

### 1.b. Ask patient the month and their age

| | |
|---|---|
| 0 | Answers both correctly |
| 1 | Answers one correctly |
| 2 | Both incorrect |

### 1.c. Ask patient to open and close eyes

| | |
|---|---|
| 0 | Obeys both correctly |
| 1 | Obeys one correctly |
| 2 | Both incorrect |

### 2. Best gaze (only horizontal eye movement)

| | |
|---|---|
| 0 | Normal |
| 1 | Partial gaze palsy |
| 2 | Forced deviation |

### 3. Visual field testing

| | |
|---|---|
| 0 | No visual field loss |
| 1 | Partial hemianopia |
| 2 | Complete hemianopia |
| 3 | Bilateral hemianopia (blind, including cortical blindness) |

### 4. Facial paresis

(ask patient to show symmetric movement of teeth or raise eyebrows and close eyes tightly)

0   Normal
1   Minor paralysis (flattened nasolabial fold, asymmetry on smiling)
2   Partial paralysis (total or near total paralysis of lower face)
3   Complete paralysis of one or both sides (absence of facial movement in the upper and lower face)

### 5. Motor function—arm (right and left)

(extends arms 90 degrees (or 45 degrees) for 10 sec without drift)

0   Normal
1   Drift
2   Some effort against gravity
3   No effort against gravity
4   No movement
9   Untestable (joint fused or limb amputated)

### 6. Motor function—leg (right and left)

(hold leg 30 degrees for 5 sec)

0   Normal
1   Drift
2   Some effort against gravity
3   No effort against gravity
4   No movement
9   Untestable (joint fused or limb amputated)

### 7. Limb ataxia

0   No ataxia
1   Present in one limb
2   Present in two limbs

(*Continued*)

TABLE 9-2

## National Institutes of Health Stroke Scale for the Assessment of Neurologic Disability (*continued*)

### 8. Sensory

(use pinprick to test arms, legs, trunk, and face—compare side to side)
0   Normal
1   Mild to moderate decrease in sensation
2   Severe to total sensory loss

### 9. Best language

(describe picture, name items, read sentences)
0   No aphasia
1   Mild to moderate aphasia
2   Severe aphasia
3   Mute

### 10. Dysarthria (read several words)

0   Normal articulation
1   Mild to moderate slurring of words
2   Near unintelligible or unable to speak
9   Intubated or other physical barrier

### 11. Extinction and inattention

0   Normal
1   Inattention or extinction to bilateral simultaneous stimulation in one
    of the sensory modalities
2   Severe hemi-inattention or hemi-inattention to more than one
    modality

(*Modified from NIH-stroke scale, revised October 2003. Full version accessible at*
*http://www.ninds.nih.gov/doctors/NIHStroke_Scale.pdf.*)

## Delirium and Dementia

Both delirium and dementia are the result of impairments in brain capacity. Delirium is the transient disorder of consciousness (acute confusional state), and dementia is the chronic decline in mental capacity. Delirium is secondary to another underlying cause and is usually reversible once the cause is identified. Major causes of delirium include infection, hypoxia, medications/drugs, and metabolic disorders. Delirium can be potentially fatal because of the underlying disorder; therefore, it is important to recognize and treat the precipitating condition quickly. Dementia is usually irreversible (except normal pressure hydrocephalus) and is commonly the result of Alzheimer disease, vascular dementia, or alcohol use.

### Pertinent Positives/Negatives: OPQRST

■ **O**nset: when and how symptoms began

■ **P**rovocative/Palliative: worsens with medication noncompliance, withdrawal; improves with time of day, medications, environment, alcohol

■ **Q**uality: history of mental status changes or "acting differently," medical history (HIV, thyroid, heart, DM, kidney, liver, genetic disorders)

■ **R**egion/**R**adiation: headache, chest pain or discomfort, dyspnea, abdominal pain, urinary symptoms

■ **S**everity: 1 to 10

■ **T**iming: constant or intermittent symptoms

Associated features: fever or chills, infections, alcohol or drug use, dialysis, social situations (nursing home, incarceration), recent traumas or falls, history of psychiatric disease, memory testing (recent and remote)

##  Physical Examination

- Fever, hypertension or hypotension, bradycardia or tachycardia, orthostatic vital signs, A&O × 3, AMS or confusion, "responding to internal stimuli," fluctuating levels of consciousness, easily distracted, incoherence, inappropriate behavior, agitated or obtunded behavior, depression, paranoia, evidence of liver disease, drug markings, tattoos, evidence of trauma, nuchal rigidity, icteric appearance, hydration status (moist mucous membranes, axillary sweat, tenting of skin), abdominal tenderness, CVA tenderness, cyanosis
- Pupillary examination
- Folstein MMSE

## Laboratory Studies

- Pulse oximetry, Accu-Chek, CBC, CMP, ECG, UA
- Consider ABG, LP, CXR, head CT, UDS, BAL

## Management

- ABCs, correct hypovolemia and electrolyte disorders
- Treat underlying cause
- Give antipsychotics/benzodiazepines for agitation and/or sedation

## Intracranial Hemorrhages (ICHs)

There are three types of ICHs: SAH, SDH, and EDH. Each entity has a high mortality rate (SAH >35%; SDH >20%–50%; EDH: >40%), so one must have a low threshold for evaluation of an ICH. SAHs result from a ruptured aneurysm or an AVM (usually a congenital berry aneurysm) and are usually described as the "worst headache of my life." SDHs result from the rupture of the bridging veins (due to a fall) and are more common in the elderly or in chronic alcoholics. EDHs result from an arterial bleed (usually the middle meningeal artery) and are associated with a trauma to the head (blunt trauma).

### Causes of Subarachnoid Hemorrhage: BATS

**B**erry aneurysm
**A**rteriovenous malformation/**A**dult polycystic kidney disease
**T**rauma (e.g., being struck with baseball **bat**)
**S**troke

## Pertinent Positives/Negatives: OPQRST

- **O**nset: when and how symptoms began
- **P**rovocative/**P**alliative: not applicable
- **Q**uality: chronic headaches, photophobia, visual changes, personality changes, AMS or confusion, "worst headache of my life"
- **R**egion/**R**adiation: headache, neck pain, bruising or bleeding, motor weakness and sensory deficits, back pain, family history of "brain bleeds"
- **S**everity: 1 to 10
- **T**iming: constant or intermittent symptoms

Associated features: trauma, falls, head injury, alcohol and/or drug use, medications, seizure, syncope, dizziness, orthostatic vital signs, bleeding disorders, nausea and/or vomiting, lethargy, neck pain or stiffness, low back pain, bilateral leg pain, history of AVM, warfarin, ASA, or heparin use, liver disease

## Physical Examination

■ Tachycardia or bradycardia, hypotension or hypertension, bradypnea or tachypnea, fever, orthostatic vital signs

■ AMS, coma, confusion; GCS (fluctuating, stable; see Table 9-1); evidence of trauma (stepoffs, bleeding, contusions, abrasions); "lucid intervals"; motor or sensory deficits; nuchal rigidity; seizures; defensive fall injuries

■ Papillary examination (fixed/dilated, sluggish)

■ Cranial nerve examination (deficiencies in cranial nerve testing)

## Laboratory Studies

■ CT, CBC, CMP, cardiac enzymes, UA, PT/PTT/INR, LP

■ Consider angiography

## Management

■ ABCs, control BP and seizures

■ Consider neurosurgical evaluation for decompression.

## Pearls

■ Cushing response (ICH): bradycardia, hypertension, bradypnea, increased ICP

■ In SAH, from 3% to 7% of all head CTs may be read as normal; therefore, it should be followed with a LP.

■ Xanthochromia is the yellowish CSF due to the breakdown of RBCs and is likely to be due to SAH rather than traumatic LP.

■ The "lucid interval" of EDH can range from several minutes to hours, followed by a dramatic change in clinical condition.

▪ ICHs on CT:
  ▪ SAH: blood in subarachnoid space
  ▪ SDH: crescent-shaped
  ▪ EDH: convex, lens-shaped

## Meningitis

Meningitis is the infection and subsequent inflammation of the leptomeninges surrounding the brain and spinal cord. Meningitis can be divided into acute (less than 24 hours), subacute (1–7 days), and chronic (more than 7 days). Acute meningitis is almost always of bacterial origin, and these patients can decompensate quickly. Bacteria enter the CNS likely via hematogenous seeding, with subsequent inflammation and edema causing increased ICP. A high index of suspicion should be maintained in patients presenting with symptoms of meningitis, because the mortality can be as high as 90%.

### Pertinent Positives/Negatives: OPQRST

▪ **O**nset: when and how symptoms began
▪ **P**rovocative/**P**alliative: worsens with light (photophobia), sound, neck movement, vomiting
▪ **Q**uality: headache and/or neck pain, AMS or confusion, acute or chronic sinus infections/ear infections, recent outbreak in community (college, military)
▪ **R**egion/**R**adiation: seizures, focal neurologic deficits
▪ **S**everity: 1 to 10
▪ **T**iming: chronic or intermittent symptoms

Associated features: fevers, chills, nuchal rigidity, nausea and/or vomiting, malaise or weakness, weight loss, night sweats, immunosuppression (DM, HIV, chemotherapy), sick contacts, recent neurosurgical procedures, splenectomy, IV drug use

 **Physical Examination**

- Fever, tachycardia or bradycardia, hypotension or hypertension, Cushing response, confused or A&O, nuchal rigidity
- Kernig sign: pain with passive extension of knee in supine patient with hip flexed
- Brudzinski sign: passive flexion of neck causes flexion of hips
- Papilledema, bulging fontanelle, focal neurologic deficits, evidence of local ENT infection (otitis media, sinusitis, mastoiditis), evidence of systemic infection (UTI, pneumonia, cellulitis), irritability, cutaneous evidence of *Neisseria meningitides* (petechiae, cutaneous hemorrhages)
- Cranial nerve examination

 **Laboratory Studies**

- Head CT, CBC, CMP, UA
- LP (with cell count, Gram stain, glucose, protein, directogens; Table 9-3)

**Management**

- Treat depending on etiology
  - In adults, ceftriaxone is the mainstay.
  - In penicillin-allergic patients, use vancomycin/gentamicin/rifampin.
- Do not delay antibiotics for LP/head CT results if meningitis is suspected.

### TABLE 9-3

## Cerebrospinal Fluid Characteristics in Bacterial and Viral Meningitis

| Parameters | Bacterial Meningitis | Viral Meningitis |
|---|---|---|
| Opening pressure | >300 mm Hg | <200 mm Hg |
| WBC | >1000/microliter | <1000/microliter |
| Differential | >80% polymorphonuclear | <50% polymorphonuclear |
| Glucose | <40 mg/dL | >40 mg/dL |
| Protein | >200 mg/dL | <200 mg/dL |
| Gram stain | Positive | Negative |
| Culture | Positive | Negative |

(*From Mick N, et al., Blueprints Emergency Medicine, 2nd ed.Blackwell Publishing 2006:126.*)

### ❌ Pearls

■ *Streptococcus pneumoniae, N. meningitides,* and *Haemophilus influenzae* are the most common organisms in bacterial meningitis.

■ In HIV-positive patients, consider herpes simplex virus, TB, and *Cryptococcus*.

## Seizure Disorder

Seizures occur with abnormal electrical discharge of neurons, resulting in focal or general neurologic symptoms. Seizures may be classified into multiple types, but two easy classifications are *generalized* (accompanied by LOC, absence, or tonic-clonic) and *partial* (focal area of abnormal electrical discharge). Seizure

### TABLE 9-4
## Differential Diagnosis of Seizure Disorder

In infants: fever/infections, primary epilepsy, trauma, tumor, metabolic (hypoglycemia, hyponatremia), developmental (AVM), hereditary, trauma, idiopathic

In adults: primary epilepsy, trauma, metabolic (hypoglycemia, hyponatremia, hypernatremia, uremia, hepatic failure), intracranial hemorrhage, AVM, masses (primary or metastatic), infectious (meningitis, abscess, encephalitis, toxoplasmosis, cysticercosis), toxins/drugs, eclampsia

disorders may be primary, but in the patient without a history of epilepsy, other causes should be investigated. In adults, trauma, stroke, metabolic disorders, alcoholism, and space-occupying lesion are the main causes of seizures. The differential diagnosis of seizures is presented in Table 9-4. Status epilepticus is prolonged seizure activity that lasts longer than 5 minutes.

### Pertinent Positives/Negatives: OPQRST

- **O**nset: when and how symptoms began, inquire about witnesses and obtain a detailed history of episode
- **P**rovocative/**P**alliative: worsens with alcohol/medication withdrawal, noncompliance with seizure medications, new medications
- **Q**uality: prodromal sensation (smell or fear), trauma prior to seizure, recollection of event, positive LOC (gradual?), change in vision, associated injuries, postictal confusion or disorientation, muscle activity
- **R**egion/**R**adiation: headache, neck, chest, or back pain
- **S**everity: 1 to 10
- **T**iming: constant or intermittent symptoms (Is this typical of your normal seizure?)

Associated features: medical history, cardiac history, DM, trauma, falls, medications, residual weakness or motor deficits, confusion, alcohol or drugs, fevers, symptoms of infection, headaches (chronic vs. acute), pregnancy

 **Physical Examination**

■ Fever, hypotension or hypertension, bradycardia or tachycardia

■ AMS, A&O, evidence of head trauma, hemotympanum, ecchymosis, tongue lacerations, bowel or urinary incontinence, neurologic deficits, cyanosis, muscle aches, shoulder dislocations, evidence of infection, nuchal rigidity

■ Cranial nerve examination (deficiencies in cranial nerve testing)

 **Laboratory Studies**

■ Accu-Chek, CBC, CMP, PT/PTT/INR, UA, β-hCG

■ Consider UDS, BAL, prolactin, head CT, anticonvulsant medication drug levels

 **Management**

■ ABCs, prevention of injury; benzodiazepines for actively seizing patients (Table 9-5)

■ Correct metabolic derangements

■ Treat underlying cause of seizure

**Treatment for Status Epilepticus: Thank Goodness All Cerebral Bursts Dissipate**

**T**hiamine
**G**lucose
**A**tivan
**C**erebyx
**B**arbiturate
**D**iprivan

**TABLE 9-5**

**Treatment of Active Seizures in the Emergency Department**

| | |
|---|---|
| **First-line agents** | |
| 1 | Benzodiazepines (midazolam, lorazepam, diazepam) |
| 2 | Short-acting barbiturates (phenobarbital, thiopental) |
| **Second-line agents** | |
| 1 | Phenytoin/fosphenytoin |
| 2 | Magnesium (for seizures thought to be due to eclampsia) |
| 3 | Valproate |
| **Refractory status epilepticus** | |
| 1 | Pentobarbital infusion (so-called pentobarbital coma) |
| 2 | Isoflurane anesthesia |

*(From Mick N, et al., Blueprints Emergency Medicine, 2nd ed. Malden, MA: Blackwell Publishin, 2006:129.)*

## Pearls

- Be aware of Todd paralysis, which is the focal neurologic deficit after a seizure.
- Seizures can cause *posterior* shoulder dislocations.
- Be aware that syncope can cause jerking movements as well (often confuses witnesses), but syncope is characterized by an immediate return to lucidity.
- A tongue laceration is almost 100% specific for a generalized seizure.

# Ophthalmology System

---

## Evaluation of Acute Vision Loss/Change

Acute vision loss/change may present for a few seconds, minutes, or hours, and is a common complaint among patients of all ages. Patients may describe a complete "black out" of their vision (monocularly or binocularly), a dimming of a certain field of vision, a "shade being pulled down" (amaurosis fugax), or a blurring or fogging effect. Ischemia is the most common cause of acute vision loss, and it may present in varying degrees of visual changes. It is best to separate causes of acute vision loss into vision loss with pain, or vision loss with no or minimal pain.

### Pertinent Positives/Negatives: OPQRST

- **O**nset: time when vision loss began, what patient was doing when it happened (e.g., walking into a dark theater [AACG], hitting head on counter [retinal detachment]), length of time symptoms lasted, whether patient has had these symptoms before

- **P**rovocative/**P**alliative: factors that make the symptoms better or worse

- **Q**uality: description of loss/change in vision (complete blackout, peripheral visual field loss, floaters/flashing lights)

- **R**egion/**R**adiation: possible associated headache, neck, back, face or ear pain

■ **S**everity: visual change in one eye or both?

■ **T**iming: constant or intermittent

Miscellaneous: trauma, past visual acuity (need for corrective lenses), previous ophthalmologic conditions (glaucoma), diabetes, atherosclerosis (especially carotid disease), high cholesterol, heart disease, AF, bleeding/clotting disorders, medication use (quinidine or Viagra), history of cancer, collagen vascular diseases, psychiatric history, photophobia, nausea, vomiting

 **Physical Examination**

■ Visual acuity in both eyes (Fig. 10-1)

■ Light/movement perception, visual fields, eyelid inflammation, pupillary dilation/constriction/accommodation, APD, extraocular muscle examination, slit lamp examination, fundus (vitreous hemorrhage), IOP, fluorescein staining

 **Laboratory Studies**

■ Consider CBC and coagulation studies

■ Consider ESR (for temporal arteritis), CT/MRI of brain, carotid imaging

**Management**

■ Treat the underlying cause

■ For ischemic causes, consider aspirin (to reduce risk of stroke) and carotid endarterectomy

**Pearls**

■ Differential diagnosis:

■ Painful causes of acute vision loss: AACG, iritis, temporal arteritis, corneal ulcer, ophthalmic migraines, ruptured globe

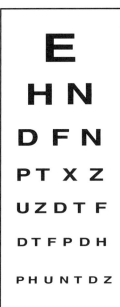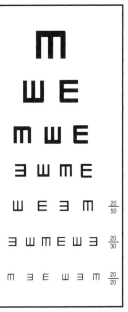

**Figure 10-1** Understanding and Using Vision Charts. Used to test distant visual acuity, the Snellen chart consists of lines of different letters stacked one on top of the other. The letters are large at the top and decrease in size from top to bottom. The chart is placed on a wall or door at eye level in a well-lighted area. The patient stands 20 feet from the chart and covers one eye with an opaque card (which prevents the patient from peeking through the fingers). Then, the patient reads each line of letters until he or she can no longer distinguish them. If the patient cannot read or has a handicap that prevents verbal communication, the E chart is used. The E chart is configured just like the Snellen chart, but the characters on it are only Es, which face in all directions. The patient is asked to indicate by pointing which way the open side of the E faces. If the patient wears glasses, they should be left on, unless they are reading glasses (reading glasses blur distance vision). (*From Weber J and Kelley J. Health Assessment in Nursing, 2nd ed. Philadelphia: Lippincott Williams & Wilkins, 2003.*)

- Painless (or minimally painful) causes of acute vision loss: cerebral ischemia (usually occlusive carotid artery disease), central retinal artery occlusion, central retinal vein occlusion, vitreous hemorrhage, retinal detachment, optic neuritis

- Optic neuritis: painful vision loss caused by inflammation of the optic nerve; strongly associated with multiple sclerosis (30% long-term risk)

- APD: to indicate an optic nerve disorder, use the "swinging flashlight test." An affected pupil dilates to a light source (Marcus Gunn pupil).

- "La belle indifférence": lack of concern for the current situation or recovery and can be seen in cases of malingering. "La belle indifférence" applies to all cases of malingering, but especially conversion blindness.

## Evaluation of the Red Eye

A red eye is extremely unnerving to the patient, and causes range from completely benign without medical intervention to high morbidity conditions. Common causes are subconjunctival hemorrhage, iritis, conjunctivitis, corneal trauma, and glaucoma. A thorough history and physical examination should reveal the underlying cause.

### Pertinent Positives/Negatives: OPQRST

- **O**nset: time that the patient noticed that his/her eye became red, whether patient has had red eye before, what the patient was doing when he/she noticed the symptoms

- **P**rovocative/**P**alliative: factors that make the eye better or worse

■ **Q**uality: feeling in eye (foreign body sensation?)

■ **R**egion/**R**adiation: possible headache, vision loss, nausea, vomiting, facial pain, eye discharge (clear or colored), eye crusting

■ **S**everity: degree of pain, bilateral or unilateral?

■ **T**iming: constant or intermittent symptoms

Miscellaneous: recent trauma (metal work), contact lenses (extended wear, daily use, overnight), photophobia, sick contacts with same condition, recent visit to eye doctor, eye surgeries, collagen vascular disease, diabetes, eye drops/medications

 **Physical Examination**

■ Visual acuity (see Figure 10-1)

■ Pupil examination (reactivity, accommodation, shape, anisocoria), external eye (periorbital skin, ptosis, subcutaneous emphysema, rashes, evidence of discharge/crusting, swelling of puncta), visual field confrontation, extraocular muscles, slit lamp examination (cells, flare, hyphema, foreign body), fluorescein dye examination (corneal uptake), papilledema, vitreous hemorrhage, IOP

 **Laboratory Studies: usually not required**

 **Management**

■ Treat underlying cause

 **Pearls**

■ Differential diagnosis: conjunctivitis, acute glaucoma, iritis, corneal abrasion, corneal ulcer, foreign body, blepharitis, cellulitis (orbital/preseptal), chalazion, hordeolum, pterygium, dacryocystitis, endophthalmitis, herpes simplex, herpes zoster

- Viral conjunctivitis: tender enlarged preauricular lymph nodes, usually clear drainage
- Bacterial conjunctivitis: usually purulent discharge
- Narrow angle glaucoma (AACG): severely painful red eye, usually older, "Asian male walked into a dark theater," pupil mid-dilated, fixed, smoky cornea, injected sclera. IOP usually greater than 30 mm Hg (>50 mm Hg not uncommon). Treat with a beta-blocker, alpha-agonist, acetazolamide, mannitol, or pilocarpine.
- Subconjunctival hemorrhage: flat, thin hemorrhage usually associated with vomiting or trauma (but can be spontaneous), benign

# 11 Musculoskeletal System

## Compartment Syndrome

Compartment syndrome is the potentially limb-threatening or life-threatening condition in which the pressure in a compartment (a closed anatomic space) exceeds the arterial perfusion pressures. The excess compartment pressure can cause tissue and muscle necrosis, ischemia, and subsequent renal failure from myoglobinuria. Major risk factors for compartment syndrome are crush injuries, edema, circumferential burns, constrictive devices, vigorous exercise, and hemorrhage. The most commonly affected compartments are in the lower extremity, but compartment syndrome can occur in the hand, forearm, buttock, thigh, leg, and foot (Table 11-1). Patients "classically" present with pain out of proportion to the injury and pain with passive flexion.

### Pertinent Positives/Negatives: OPQRST

- **O**nset: when and how symptoms began
- **P**rovocative/**P**alliative: worsens with active or passive movement; improves with fasciotomy
- **Q**uality: pain: pressure, achy, burning, "pain out of proportion to examination"
- **R**egion/**R**adiation: pain restricted to one extremity?
- **S**everity: 1 to 10
- **T**iming: constant or intermittent pain

## TABLE 11-1

### Common Sites and Etiologies of Compartment Syndrome

| Location | Etiology |
| --- | --- |
| Lower leg | Tibia fractures |
| Forearm | Supracondylar humerus fractures |
| Foot | Calcaneus fracture |
| Thigh | Crush |
| Hand | Crush |

(*From NMS Surgery, 4th ed. Jarrell BE, Carabasi RA III, Rado JS [eds.]. Philadelphia: Lippincott Williams & Wilkins, 2000;565.*)

Associated features: trauma (MVA, crush injury, burn, hemorrhaging); numbness, tingling, or paresthesias; use of constrictive devices (tight clothing, casts/splints); limb fractures; exercise (especially overuse); recent surgery; recent burn injury; dyspnea; limb swelling; vascular puncture

 **Physical Examination**

■ "Pain out of proportion to the injury"
■ Pain with passive flexion, peripheral pulses, change in skin temperature/cold extremity, evidence of DVT, obvious bone deformity, burns, paresthesias/hypesthesias, two point discrimination, pallor, tenseness of compartment, evidence of focal deficits, use of anticoagulants

**Laboratory Studies**

■ Measurement of compartment pressure
■ Plain film x-ray

### 💊 Management

■ Fasciotomy (if pressures >30 mm Hg)

### ✳ Pearls

■ Patients with AMS may not be able to report compartmental pain.

**6 Ps** of compartment syndrome:

**P**ain
**P**aresthesias
**P**aralysis
**P**oikilothermia
**P**ulselessness (very late sign)
**P**allor

## Deep Vein Thrombosis (DVT)

DVTs are thrombi that generally form in the lower extremity in the calf veins, near the valve cusps. Virchow angle (stasis, hypercoagulability, vessel wall injury) is often used to explain the formation of a DVT. Stasis results from immobilization (surgery, long trips, bed rest), hypercoagulability results from procoagulant factors (antithrombin III, protein C or S deficiency), and vessel wall injury results from surgery or catheterization (IV lines). The majority of DVTs dissolve spontaneously; however, up to 20% may propagate and "embolize" to the pulmonary vasculature, resulting in a pulmonary embolism. Patients with DVTs may often be asymptomatic, and a high index of suspicion is necessary in hospitalized patients.

## Pertinent Positives/Negatives: OPQRST

■ **O**nset: when and how symptoms began; sudden onset of pain?

■ **P**rovocative/**P**alliative: worsens with ambulation, palpation; may improve with elevation

■ **Q**uality: thigh, leg, or arm pain; aching, pressure, sharp, or burning pain

■ **R**egion/**R**adiation: chest, back, neck, or abdominal pain; possible dyspnea

■ **S**everity: 1 to 10

■ **T**iming: constant or intermittent pain

Associated features: fever or chills, history of DVTs or blood clots, family history of DVT, recent surgery or trauma, central line, recent immobilization (bed rest or travel), malignancy, IV drug use, oral contraceptives, obesity, age (>40 years), erythema, tenderness, swelling, orthopedic injury, pregnancy/postpartum, CHF, renal disease, HIV, autoimmune diseases, paresthesias

## Physical Examination

■ Fever, tachycardia, hypertension

■ Erythema/tenderness/swelling to extremity, Homans sign, palpable cords, cyanosis, peripheral pulses, capillary refill, recent surgical scars, evidence of IV drug use, abdominal ecchymosis from LMWH, distended veins, chest tenderness, edema

■ Measure lower extremities (compare to other side)

## Laboratory Studies

■ D-dimer, U/S of extremities, PT/PTT/INR

■ Consider x-ray, ABI, protein C/S, factor V Leiden, antithrombin III

### 💊 Management

■ Anticoagulation (heparin vs. LMWH)
■ Consider Greenfield filter if patient is unable to take anticoagulants

### ❋ Pearls

■ Homans sign: pain on dorsiflexion of the foot; an unspecific and insensitive finding
■ Phlegmasia cerulea dolens: discoloration due to DVT, often red/purple
■ Phlegmasia alba dolens: massive ileofemoral venous thrombosis with associated arterial spasm; pale, pulseless extremities

## Evaluation of Orthopedic Injuries (Fracture Terminology)

There are multiple types of fractures, and these should be classified on presentation. "Typical" fractures result from trauma to healthy bone. Pathologic fractures result from a minimal insult to diseased or abnormal bone (i.e., metastatic lesions, bone cysts, osteoporosis). Epiphyseal (Salter-Harris) fractures involve the epiphyseal plate near the ends of long bones of growing children and adolescents (Fig. 11-1). When describing the radiographic appearance of a fracture, one should explain the pathology so that the listener can visualize the fracture as he or she hears the report.

Fractures can be described in terms of the following characteristics:

■ Open vs. closed: open fractures are considered orthopedic emergencies that require IV antibiotics and a washout in the OR.

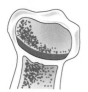
a.) Separation at physis

b.) Separation at physis with partial metaphyseal fracture

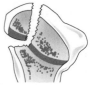
c.) Partial separation at physis with intra-articular epiphyseal fracture

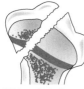
d.) Intra-articular fracture extending across physis into metaphysis

e.) Compression or crush of physis

a.) **S**eparation
b.) **A**bove
c.) **L**ower
d.) **T**hrough
e.) **E**verything
   **R**uined

**Figure 11-1** Salter-Harris Classification of Fractures. Class b fractures are the most common, and class e fractures have the worst prognosis. (*From Mick N, et al., Blueprints Emergency Medicine, 2nd ed. Malden, MA: Blackwell Publishing, 2006:86.*)

- Location of fracture: proximal, distal, middle third; note if there is an intra-articular fracture.
- Orientation of fracture line: comminuted, transverse, oblique, greenstick, spiral, segmental, torus
- Displacement: Are the fracture fragments offset from each other?
- Angulation: direction of angulation and amount (degrees)

## Osteomyelitis

Osteomyelitis is the infection of bone and surrounding tissues. It results from either hematogenous seeding/spread (20%) or soft tissue infection (80%). Osteomyelitis can be classified as acute (no previous bone infection), subacute (Brodie abscess), or chronic (failed treatment or untreated osteomyelitis). Hematogenous spread is more common in children and IV drug users. *Staphylococcus aureus* is the most common organism found in osteomyelitis.

### Pertinent Positives/Negatives: OPQRST

- **O**nset: when and how symptoms began
- **P**rovocative/**P**alliative: worsens with weight bearing, pressure, examination, ROM; may improve with surgery or antibiotics, drainage
- **Q**uality: bone and joint pain, history of previous bone infections, back and neck pain, trauma to area (puncture wound), discharge from wound
- **R**egion/**R**adiation: limited ROM in joint
- **S**everity: 1 to 10
- **T**iming: constant or intermittent symptoms

Associated features: fevers or chills, history of previous febrile illnesses, night sweats, fatigue, weakness, AMS, erythema, tenderness, diabetes, IV drug use or HIV, previous bone injury/joint replacement, sickle cell anemia

###  Physical Examination

- Fever, tachycardia, hypotension
- Discomfort, erythema, joint and bone tenderness, swelling, sinus drainage, evidence of other infection, decreased ROM, surgical or trauma scars, evidence of IV drug use, spinal tenderness, inability to bear weight

###  Laboratory Studies

- CBC, ESR/CRP, blood culture, CXR, wound culture
- Consider CT, bone scan, or MRI

### 🔖 Management

- IV antibiotics (penicillin/cephalosporin)
- Surgical débridement

### ✳ Pearls

- Osteomyelitis may not be visible on x-rays until 10–14 days later.
  - Involucrum: reactive periosteal bone growth
  - Sequestrum: localized bone necrosis
- In sickle cell anemia, think of *Salmonella*.
- In chronic wounds, it is often possible to culture *S. aureus* and *Pseudomonas*.

---

## Rheumatoid Arthritis and Osteoarthritis

---

RA is a chronic, systemic inflammatory arthritis involving the synovium and articular structures of multiple joints. The etiology of RA is still unknown, but it is likely genetic. RA is associated with joint deformity, especially in the wrists, MCP, and PIP joints, as well as with systemic symptoms such as fatigue, weight loss, and malaise. OA, the most common type of joint disease, is characterized by the destabilization of articular cartilage and subchondral bone. OA is thought to be due to "wear and tear" and overuse, but may also be secondary to joint trauma. OA often affects weight-bearing joints, such as the knees, hips, and lumbosacral spine.

### Pertinent Positives/Negatives: OPQRST

- **O**nset: when and how symptoms began; onset of pain sudden or gradual

■ **P**rovocative/**P**alliative: worsens in morning or evening, with stretching, exercising, or weight bearing; improves with warmth, medications, weight loss, few minutes of movement

■ **Q**uality: joint pain, multiple or single joints, "locking" of joints

■ **R**egion/**R**adiation: headache; neck, back, or hip pain?

■ **S**everity: 1 to 10

■ **T**iming: constant or intermittent symptoms

Associated features: obesity, occupation (for repetitive motions), duration of pain, joints affected, migratory pattern of pain, trauma or injury to joints affected, number of joints affected, weakness, malaise, weight loss, subcutaneous nodes, joint deformity, fevers, family history, hematemesis, melena, anemia

##  Physical Examination

■ Fever

■ Joint deformities (ulnar deviation, swan neck, Heberden or Bouchard nodes, boutonnière deformity), joint guarding, limited ROM, inability to bear weight, crepitus, instability, erythema, discharge, swelling, subcutaneous nodules, scleritis, dryness of eyes, scars from trauma or surgery

■ DRE with stool guaiac

##  Laboratory Studies

■ Obtain an x-ray of the involved joint

■ Consider ESR/CRP, rheumatoid factor, joint aspiration

##  Management

■ NSAIDs

■ Weight loss, physical/occupational therapy

- DMARDs (gold, hydroxychloroquine [Plaquenil], azathioprine [Imuran], MTX)

## ❊ Pearls

- OA pain is usually worse with activity and relieved with rest.
- RA presents with morning stiffness relieved with activity.
- OA affects the outer digits (Heberden nodes, DIP, Bouchard nodes, PIP).
- RA: ulnar deviation, boutonnière deformity (hyperextension of DIP, flexion of PIP), swan neck deformity (flexion of DIP, extension of PIP)

## 📖 Literature

- Wells PS, Anderson DR, Rodger M, et al. Evaluation of D-dimer in the diagnosis of suspected deep-vein thrombosis. *N Engl J Med.* 2003 Sep 25;349(13):1227–1235. Wells et al. found that DVT can be ruled out in a patient who is clinically judged unlikely to have a DVT if the patient also has a negative D-dimer.

# 12 Dermatology: Evaluation of Rashes

Most skin lesions involve either allergies (medication-induced, contact), infections (e.g., cellulitis, erysipelas), or irritants (chemical). The key to diagnosing rashes is pattern recognition, and fortunately, there are few conditions that are immediately life-threatening. Types of lesions include the following:

- Macule: flat lesion, <1 cm in diameter
- Petechia: flat, nonblanching purple spot, <2 mm in diameter
- Purpura: flat, nonblanching purple discoloration of skin
- Nodule: elevated palpable solid lesion <1 cm in diameter
- Wheal: flat/elevated edematous papule or plaque with erythema
- Vesicle: elevated, circumscribed, thin-walled blister <5 mm in diameter
- Bulla: elevated, circumscribed, thin-walled blister >5 mm in diameter
- Papule: elevated solid, palpable lesion <1 cm in diameter
- Plaque: elevated, flat topped, formed by confluence of papules >0.5 cm in diameter

## Pertinent Positives/Negatives: OPQRST (Fig. 12-1)

- **O**nset: when the patient first noticed the rash; whether the rash has stayed the same, spread, or diminished; whether the rash is generalized or localized; whether the rash comes and goes; whether the rash leave spots when it resolves

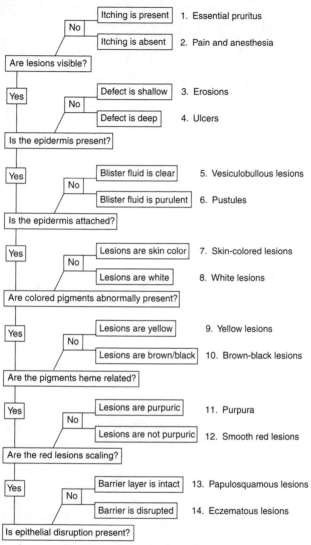

**Figure 12-1** Problem-oriented dermatologic algorithm. (*Modified from Lynch PJ, Dermatology, 3rd ed. Philadelphia: Williams & Wilkins, 1994:89–105. Reprinted with permission.*)

■ **P**rovocative/**P**alliative: factors that make the rash better, factors that make the rash worse, whether the patient has seen *any* health-care provider for this rash before

■ **Q**uality: not applicable

■ **R**egion/**R**adiation: not applicable

■ **S**everity: whether the rash is painful or pruritic (1 to 10)

■ **T**iming: constant or intermittent

Miscellaneous: fevers, chills, weakness, fatigue, duration of rash, progression, evolution of rash, similar lesions in past, distribution, involvement of mouth/anus/genitalia, history of STDs or genital discharge, medications, IV drug use, occupation, exposure to animals/insects/plants, chemical exposure, new food exposure, exposure to sun, immunization history, family history of dermatologic disorders

 **Physical Examination**

■ Fever, chills

■ Consider the distribution, extent, arrangement, pattern, blanching pattern, color, and morphology of the rash or lesion

 **Laboratory Studies**

■ Biopsy, KOH prep, culture

 **Management**

■ Treat the underlying cause.

■ Consider steroids, emollient creams/lotions, and antibiotics if indicated.

 **Pearls**

■ Rule of nines in burns: 9% arms, 18% each leg, 18% torso, 18% back, 9% head, 1% size of palm of hand (Fig. 12-2)

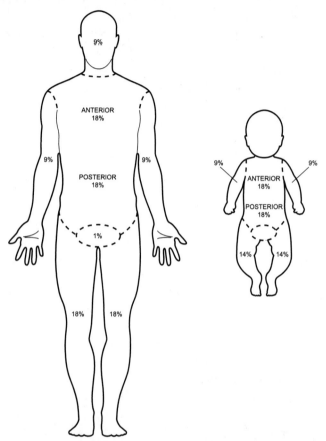

**Figure 12-2** Rule of nines. Approximate burn surface area; adult and child. (*From Mick N, et al., Blueprints Emergency Medicine, 2nd ed. Malden, MA: Blackwell Publishing, 2006:94.*)

- "If it's wet, dry it; if it's dry, wet it."
- Be aware of petechiae associated with AMS and fever for meningococcemia and Rocky Mountain spotted fever.
- Check the current medications the patient is taking; it is important to rule out a drug reaction!
- Causes of petechial rash and fever
  - Infectious: endocarditis, meningococcemia, gonococcemia, rickettsia, enterovirus, dengue fever, hepatitis B, rubella, EBV, rat bite fever, epidemic typhus
  - Noninfectious: allergy, thrombocytopenia, scurvy, lupus, Henoch-Schönlein purpura, hypersensitivity vasculitis, rheumatic fever, amyloidosis
- Causes of maculopapular rash and fever
  - Infectious: typhus, secondary syphilis, Lyme disease, meningococcemia, mycoplasma, psittacosis, rickettsia, leptospirosis, parvovirus B19, rubeola, EBV, adenovirus, primary HIV
  - Noninfectious: allergy, serum sickness, erythema multiforme, erythema marginatum, lupus, dermatomyositis
- Causes of vesiculobullous rash and fever
  - Infectious: staphylococcemia, *Gonococcus*, rickettsia, herpes, varicella, *Vibrio*, folliculitis, enterovirus, parvovirus B19, HIV
  - Noninfectious: plant dermatitis, allergy, eczema vaccinatum, erythema multiforme
- Causes of erythematous rash and fever
  - Infectious: staphylococcal/streptococcal infection (toxic shock syndrome), *Streptococcus viridans*, Kawasaki disease
  - Noninfectious: allergy, vasodilation, eczema, psoriasis, lymphoma, pityriasis rubra pilaris
- Causes of urticarial rash and fever

- Infectious: mycoplasma, Lyme disease, enterovirus, HIV, EBV, *Strongyloides*, trichinosis, schistosomiasis, loiasis
- Noninfectious: allergy, vasculitis, malignancy, idiopathic

### Literature

- Levin S, Goodman LJ. An approach to acute fever and rash (AFR) in the adult. *Curr Clin Topics Infect Dis.* 1995;15:19–75.
- Schlossberg D. Fever and rash. *Infect Dis Clin North Am.* 1996 Mar;10(1):101–110.

# Infectious Disease

## Fever

Fever is defined as a temperature of 100.4°F or greater, but be aware that a fever greater than 106.7°F is called hyperpyrexia, a distinctly different entity. Body temperature is regulated by the hypothalamus. Fever is caused by pyrogens, bacterial or viral infection, or cells undergoing autolysis. Pyrogens affect the anterior hypothalamus and reset the thermal set point above 98.6°F. Be aware that there are many causes of fever besides infectious, such as neuroleptic malignant syndrome, medication side effects (anticholinergics), hyperthyroidism, collagen vascular disease, and granulomatous disease.

### Pertinent Positives/Negatives: OPQRST

- **O**nset: when fever began, history of similar fever, what patient was doing when he or she noticed the fever, whether patient has checked fever at home on a thermometer
- **P**rovocative/**P**alliative: determine whether the fever resolves on its own, is getting better or worse, conditions that make fever better or worse, whether it is worse at a certain time of day
- **Q**uality: possible shaking rigors/chills
- **R**egion/**R**adiation: not applicable
- **S**everity: not applicable
- **T**iming: constant or intermittent

Miscellaneous: AMS, night sweats, appetite, medications (prescription and over-the-counter), surgical procedures, dental procedures, family history of febrile illnesses/collagen vascular diseases, exposure to TB, HIV-positive status, IV drug use, hemoglobinopathies, occupational history, smoking, rashes, recent viral illnesses, birthplace/geographic area, occupation, tick/insect bites, back pain/neck pain/headache, history of heart murmur, recent travel

## Physical Examination

- Fever, tachycardia, hypertension, hypotension, tachypnea
- A&O × 3, comfortable to toxic-appearing, rashes, cutaneous evidence of erythema/infections, malar rashes, pharyngeal erythema, dental tenderness, lymphadenopathy, IV drug use track marks, abdominal tenderness, heart murmur, genital discharge
- Pelvic examination (tenderness)
- Rectal examination (tenderness, purulent discharge)

## Laboratory Studies

- CBC, CMP, CXR, UA, BC × 2
- Consider further diagnostic imaging for localized infection (e.g., head CT), LP, CRP/ESR, ANA/RF

## Management

- Treat underlying infection if present
- Stop offending drug if "drug fever"
- Antipyretics (Tylenol, Motrin)

## Pearls

- Axillary temperatures are unreliable; repeat with oral or rectal temperature.

■ Postoperative fever:
  ■ Wind (POD 1–2): atelectasis/systemic inflammatory response
  ■ Water (POD 3–5): UTIs (Foley catheters)
  ■ Walking (POD 4–6): DVTs
  ■ Wound (POD 5–7): infections of wound/incision
  ■ Wonder drugs (POD 7+)

### Rheumatic Fever: Modified Jones Criteria–JONES CRITERIA (Major Criteria)

**J**oint (arthritis)
**O**bvious (cardiac)
**N**odule (rheumatic)
**E**rythema marginatum
**S**ydenham chorea
**(Minor Criteria)**
**I**nflammatory cells (leukocytosis)
**T**emperature (fever)
**E**SR/CRP elevated
**R**aised PR interval
**I**tself (previous history of rheumatic fever)
**A**rthralgia

## Human Immunodeficiency Virus (HIV) and Acquired Immunodeficiency Syndrome (AIDS)

HIV is the virus that causes AIDS. Acute HIV infection presents as a nonspecific flu-like presentation and can remain dormant for an average of 8 years in adults. AIDS indicator conditions occur at about a CD4 count of 500 cells/μL, and examples include oral thrush, vulvovaginal candidiasis, neuropathy, and recurrent herpes zoster. AIDS is defined as a

CD4 count of less than 200 cells/μL or the presence of an "indicator" illness, such as esophageal candidiasis, PCP, Kaposi sarcoma, or HIV encephalopathy. A strong index of suspicion should be maintained in patients with late-stage HIV/AIDS, because they may not manifest the typical signs and symptoms or the laboratory findings associated with systemic infections.

## Pertinent Positives/Negatives: OPQRST

- **O**nset: length of time patient has had HIV, patient's last CD4 count, whether patient is taking any anti-HIV medications
- **P**rovocative/**P**alliative: not applicable
- **Q**uality: patient's symptoms and length of time they have been present
- **R**egion/**R**adiation: not applicable
- **S**everity: 1 to 10
- **T**iming: constant or intermittent

Miscellaneous: latest CD4/viral load count, compliance with anti-HIV medications, fevers, chills, weakness, fatigue, appetite, weight loss, IV drug use, homosexual behavior, history of blood transfusions, hemophilia, unprotected sex, headache, neck stiffness, confusion, thrush, dysphagia, dyspnea, chest pain, cough, abdominal pain, vomiting, diarrhea, dysuria, vaginal/penile discharge, focal neurologic deficits, rash

## Physical Examination

- Fever, tachycardia, hypotension, toxic appearance, confusion/AMS
- Evidence of skin infection/erythema/Kaposi sarcoma, rales/ rhonchi, sputum, dehydration, cachexia, temporal wasting, oral candidiasis, oral hairy leukoplakia, lymphadenopathy,

focal neurologic deficits, cardiac murmur, abdominal tenderness, organomegaly
■ Pelvic examination (evidence of infection)

### Laboratory Studies
■ CBC, CMP, LDH (for PCP), ABG (for PCP), BC × 2, stool/urine cultures, CXR, UA
■ Consider LP, head CT, HIV antibodies, CD4 count, viral load

### Management
■ ABCs
■ Correct hypovolemia
■ Empiric antibiotics for presenting infection

### Pearls
■ Meningismus is frequently absent in cryptococcal meningitis
■ Opportunistic infections occur with a CD4 count of less than 200 cells/µL
■ Recipients of blood products between the years 1975 and 1985 may have been exposed to HIV in the blood products.
■ Up to 25% of patients with PCP may have a normal CXR.

## Septic Shock

Sepsis is a vast syndrome caused by any type of microorganism (bacteria, fungi, mycobacteria, virus, rickettsia). Initially, the body responds with SIRS, which includes fever, tachypnea, tachycardia, and leukocytosis (Table 13-1). If SIRS is present with a documented infection (bacteremia), it is considered sepsis. Severe sepsis is sepsis resulting in end-organ damage or hypoperfusion. Septic shock is severe sepsis with hypotension despite fluid resuscitation. The most frequent sites of infection are the lungs, abdomen, and urinary tract. Sepsis should be suspected early, because the mortality for septic shock approaches 50%.

### Pertinent Positives/Negatives: OPQRST

- **O**nset: length of time the patient has been feeling ill, when the illness began, the initial symptom, any previous history of such feelings

### TABLE 13-1

#### Cardiac Parameters and Formulas

Cardiac output (CO) = Heart rate × Stroke volume (normal, 4–8 L/min)

Cardiac index (CI) = CO/Body Surface Area (normal, 2.8–4.2 L/min/m$^2$)

Mean arterial pressure (MAP) = 1/3 systolic BP + 2/3 diastolic BP (normal, 80–100 mm Hg)

Systemic vascular resistance (SVR) = (MAP – CVP) × (80)/CO (normal, 800–1100 dynes/sec/cm$^2$)

Pulmonary vascular resistance (PVR) = (Pulmonary artery pressure, mean [PAM] – Pulmonary capillary wedge pressure [PCWP])(80)/CO (normal, 45–120 dynes/sec/cm$^2$)

Central venous pressure (CVP) = (normal, 8–12 cm H$_2$O)

Pulmonary artery systolic pressure = (normal, 20–30 mm Hg)

Pulmonary artery diastolic pressure = (normal, 10–15 mm Hg)

Pulmonary artery mean pressure = (15–20 mm Hg)

Pulmonary capillary wedge pressure (PCWP, or "wedge pressure") = (normal, 8–12 mm Hg)

■ **P**rovocative/**P**alliative: not applicable
■ **Q**uality: not applicable
■ **R**egion/**R**adiation: not applicable
■ **S**everity: not applicable
■ **T**iming: constant or intermittent

Miscellaneous (most often to find cause of sepsis): fevers, chills, fatigue, malaise, confusion, anxiety, agitation, underlying medical conditions (DM, HIV, cirrhosis), medications, fever onset, $T_{max}$, diaphoresis, headache, neck stiffness, dysphagia, appetite, dental pain, ear pain, skin erythema, joint pain, IV drug use, cough, pleuritic chest pain, abdominal pain, nausea, vomiting, diarrhea, dysuria, pregnancy, vaginal discharge, trauma, recent antibiotic use (past 3 months), recent surgery (especially prosthetics)

 **Physical Examination**

■ Fever, hypothermia (especially in elderly or immunocompromised), tachycardia, tachypnea, toxic appearance
■ AMS, cool skin, diaphoretic, dry mucous membranes, meningismus, inflamed tympanic membranes, pharyngeal erythema/exudates, swollen tonsils, lymphadenopathy, rales/rhonchi, murmur (especially new), abdominal pain, CVA tenderness
■ Suprapubic tenderness, tenderness on pelvic examination (cervical motion/adnexal tenderness), retained foreign body

 **Laboratory Studies**

■ CBC with differential, CMP, LFTs, ABG, PT/PTT, D-dimer, UA, urine culture, BC × 2, CXR
■ Consider CT, U/S, CRP, LP

TABLE 13-2

## Vasopressors Used in the Management of Shock

| Agent (typical dosages) | β-1 | β-2 | α-1 |
| --- | --- | --- | --- |
| Isoproterenol (0.01–0.1 µg/kg/min) | +++ | +++ | 0 |
| Norepinephrine (0.05–1 µg/kg/min) | ++ | 0 | +++ |
| Epinephrine (0.05–2 µg/kg/min) | +++ | ++ | +++ |
| Phenylephrine (0.5–5 µg/kg/min) | 0 | 0 | +++ |
| Dopamine* (1–20 µg/kg/min) | +(++) | + | +(++) |
| Dobutamine (2.5–20 µg/kg/min) | +++ | + | + |

*Dopamine effects at "high dose," which are typically greater than 3 to 5 µg/kg/min, are shown in parentheses. 0, no effect; +, minimal effect; ++, moderate effect; +++, substantial effect.

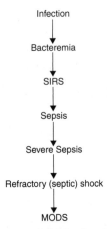

**Figure 13-1** Development of shock, showing that it is on a continuum. MODS = multiple organ dysfunction syndrome; SIRS = systemic inflammatory response syndrome.

## 🔖 Management (Table 13-2)

■ ABCs, intubation if necessary

■ Aggressive fluid resuscitation with possible adrenergic agents

■ Empiric antibiotics, surgical intervention if necessary

■ Antipyretics

## ✳️ Pearls

■ Septic shock is on a continuum (Fig. 13-1)

■ SIRS: temperature >100.4°F or <96.8°C, heart rate >90 beats/min, respiratory rate >20 breaths/min or $PaCO_2$ <32 mm Hg, leukocytosis >12,000/(L or >10%) bands. Be aware that tachycardia may not be present in the elderly or in patients taking beta-blockers.

# 14 Toxicology/Overdose

Many times a drug overdose is intentional, but it is important to remember that not all overdoses are a result of suicidal ideation. Many patients, especially at the "extremes of age," may present with accidental drug ingestions, or cases of medication error may present as an overdose. Although all chemicals are potentially poisonous, and each has its own specific treatment, a basic management can be used for almost all overdoses. It is important to stabilize and maintain the ABCs and manage an abnormal BP or heart rate. Next, it is necessary to search for a specific toxidrome, that is, a constellation of signs and symptoms particular to a substance. Once identified, diagnostic workup and appropriate treatment may proceed.

## Pertinent Positives/Negatives: OPQRST

- **O**nset: time of ingestion/exposure, previous use of ingested substances (acute vs. chronic ingestion)
- **P**rovocative/**P**alliative: suicidal ideations, previous suicide attempts, presence of suicide note
- **Q**uality: not applicable
- **R**egion/**R**adiation: not applicable
- **S**everity: not applicable
- **T**iming: not applicable

Miscellaneous: paramedic/emergency medical services report of scene and medications/pills/prescriptions, number of pills ingested, accidental ingestion, occupation of patient, AMS,

| **TABLE 14-1** |
| --- |
| Characteristic Findings of Drug Overdose |

Heroin
- Miosis (pinpoint pupils)
- Respiratory depression
- Bradycardia
- Depressed level of consciousness

Cocaine
- Mydriasis (dilated pupils)
- Tachycardia
- Hypertension
- Euphoria/central nervous system excitation
- Hyperthermia

Amphetamines
- Mydriasis
- Tachycardia
- Hypertension
- Insomnia
- Anorexia
- Psychosis

*(From Mick N, et al., Blueprints Emergency Medicine, 2nd ed. Malden, MA: Blackwell Publishing, 2006:193.)*

chest pain, lethargy, seizures, visual changes, diarrhea, nausea/vomiting, fevers, abdominal pain, palpitations, alcohol use, drug use, smoking, medical illnesses

## Physical Examination (Table 14-1)

■ Fever, tachycardia or bradycardia, hypotension or hypertension, bradypnea or tachypnea

■ AMS, agitation, confusion, slurred speech, ataxia, nystagmus, pinpoint/dilated pupils, dysconjugate gaze, lacrimation,

**TABLE 14-2**

## Quick Guide to Overdoses

| Overdosed Substance | Antidote/Treatment |
|---|---|
| Opioids (heroin, morphine, acetaminophen/oxycodone [Percocet]) | Narcan |
| Cholinergics (organophosphates) | Atropine, 2-pralidoxime (2-PAM) |
| Anticholinergics (atropine, scopolamine) | Physostigmine |
| Hypoglycemia (insulin, oral hypoglycemics) | Glucose |
| Sympathomimetics (cocaine, amphetamines) | Benzodiazepines |
| Benzodiazepines | Flumazenil (with caution for seizures) |
| Aspirin/salicylates | Urine alkalinization |
| Digoxin | Digibind |
| Acetaminophen | Acetylcysteine (Mucomyst) |
| Calcium channel blockers | IV calcium, insulin |
| Beta blockers | Glucagon |
| Tricyclic antidepressants | Urine alkalinization |
| Lithium | Sodium polystyrene sulfonate (Kayexalate), hemodialysis |
| Ethylene glycol | Ethanol/fomepizole |

dry mouth, salivation, cyanosis, flushing, evidence of trauma, IV drug track marks, bowel sounds, abdominal tenderness

■ Evidence of previous suicide attempts (lacerations to wrists)

### 🔬 Laboratory Studies

■ CMP, LFTs, PT/INR, anion gap, Accu-Chek, ABG, drug screen, ethanol level, CXR, ECG, UA, β-hCG

■ Specific toxin identifier (phenytoin, iron, acetaminophen)

### 💊 Management

■ ABCs, correct hypovolemia, electrolyte imbalance

■ Initial management includes a "coma cocktail": **DON'T: D**extrose, **O**xygen, **N**arcan, **T**hiamine

■ Treat for specific ingestion

■ Consider lavage if ingestion within 1 hour, activated charcoal (for all except hydrocarbons, acids/alkalis/alcohols, iron, lithium) with sorbitol, urinary alkalinization, hemodialysis (ASA, lithium, ethylene glycol, barbiturates, theophylline), whole bowel irrigation

### ✳️ Pearls

■ Assume that all prescriptions were "full" at the time of ingestion; therefore if 10 pills are missing from a bottle of 30, then all 10 pills were ingested recently.

■ See Table 14-2, which is a handy guide to overdoses.

## Abdominal Pain

Although some diseases are common to both adults and children, others are age specific and can present a diagnostic challenge. The age of the patient influences the presentation and workup of the patient. The workup of a neonate with vomiting is far different from the workup of a 2-year-old with vomiting. An infant or young child is also unable to give a complete history, so when a young patient presents with pain, vomiting, diarrhea, constipation, or GI bleeding, a high index of suspicion is necessary.

### Pertinent Positives/Negatives: OPQRST

- **O**nset: length of time symptoms have been present, when the patient last felt "normal," what the child was doing before the pain began
- **P**rovocative/**P**alliative: determine what makes pain better or worse
- **Q**uality: Ask the patient to qualify the pain (he or she is usually unable to); is the patient "acting right"?
- **R**egion/**R**adiation: Determine whether the condition appears to be abdominal or extra-abdominal, obstructive or nonobstructive, or systemic or local
- **S**everity: 1 to 10
- **T**iming: intermittent or constant pain. Ask whether there are completely pain-free periods; determine "fussiness" or irritability; is a baby "grunting in pain"?

Miscellaneous: Does the child appear to be sick or healthy and happy?

Associated features: fever; abdominal masses; upper or lower GI bleeding; abdominal, flank, or rectal pain; vomiting (quality and quantity); diarrhea (qualify and quantify); constipation (normal number of bowel movements vs. number now); jaundice; bruising (Henoch-Schönlein purpura); feeding and bowel habits; appetite; hematemesis/hematochezia; medical history (prematurity, CF, sickle cell disease, inborn errors of metabolism); presence of lead in household; evidence of trauma

##  Physical Examination

■ Ill-appearing child
■ Observe movements of child (walking/interactions)
■ Fever, tachycardia, hypotension
■ AMS, hydration status (mucosa, anterior fontanelle), tender abdomen (watch child's face), hernia check, bruising/petechiae, rashes, abdominal masses (olive- or sausage-like mass), visible peristalsis, lung fields (pneumonia), testes, surgical scars
■ Rectal examination (guaiac)

## Laboratory Studies (Guided by History)

■ CBC, UA, CMP, β-hCG, lipase
■ Consider x-ray (including chest), U/S, CT

##  Management

■ Stabilize patient, fluid resuscitation, possible surgical evaluation
■ Consider antibiotics
■ Treat underlying cause

## �֎ Pearls

- Peritoneal pain is worsened by movement, so the patient may remain immobile.
- Obstructive pain is associated with restlessness and motion.
- Volvulus: life-threatening complication of malrotation, vomiting, abdominal distension, and bloody streaks in stool
- Pyloric stenosis: hypertrophy of smooth muscle that narrows antrum of stomach, projective vomiting (never bilious), and failure to gain weight. Treat with IV hydration and surgery.
- Intussusception: telescoping of bowel into another segment, sudden onset of pain, with just as sudden resolution of symptoms, "currant jelly" stool, and positive guaiac. Air contrast enema is diagnostic and often curative.
- Hirschsprung disease: absence of ganglionic cells in distal colon, resulting in intestinal obstruction, constipation, and abdominal distension. A narrowed distal colon with proximal dilation is the classic finding of Hirschsprung's disease after a barium enema.

## Child Abuse

Child abuse, often thought of as only physical abuse, should be thought of as an all-inclusive phrase, including sexual abuse, emotional abuse, neglect, and Münchhausen syndrome by proxy. The medical provider should be able to suspect abuse, recognize signs and symptoms, treat any medical conditions, report the suspected abuse to authorities, and document the findings. Each year, more than one million children suffer from abuse or neglect, and more than one thousand die as a result of abuse.

## Pertinent Positives/Negatives: OPQRST

■ **O**nset: ask the following questions:
  ■ How did the injury/condition happen?
  ■ Is the history consistent with the nature of the injury?
  ■ Was there a delay in seeking medical care?
  ■ Is there appropriate parental concern?
  ■ Are there unexplained or poorly explained injuries?
  ■ Is there a changing history?
  ■ Are the injuries compatible with the mechanism?
■ **P**rovocative/**P**alliative: not applicable
■ **Q**uality: not applicable
■ **R**egion/**R**adiation: not applicable
■ **S**everity: not applicable
■ **T**iming: not applicable

Miscellaneous: Try to interview everyone separately; ask the date of the LMP, a history of STDs, a history of previous fractures, chronic illnesses, and "bruising problems"; avoid leading questions; ask about sexual abuse, witnessed abuse, domestic violence; ask "Do you feel safe at home?"

## 📕 Physical Examination

■ Poor hygiene, poor eye contact, lethargy, persistent unexplained vomiting (head injury), seizures, apnea, coma, irritability (difficult to console), little subcutaneous tissue (skinny), occipital alopecia, abdominal pain
■ Obvious signs of trauma, obvious pattern injuries (hand mark, bite mark, iron burn; Fig. 15-1), bruises in multiple stages of healing (Table 15-1), burns, multiplanar injuries

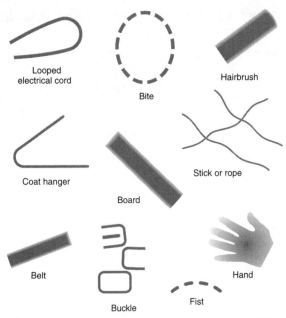

**Figure 15-1** Cutaneous findings of instruments used in child abuse. (*From Marino B, Fine K. Blueprints Pediatrics, 4th ed. Philadelphia: Lippincott Williams & Wilkins, 2007:14.*)

### Laboratory Studies

- CBC, coagulation studies (bruising), "trauma series" x-rays or skeletal surveys (all long bones, ribs, clavicles, digits, pelvis, skull), UA, liver enzymes/amylase (if abdominal trauma)
- Consider head and abdominal CT

### Management

- Stabilize patient
- Treat any medical conditions as appropriate
- Inform law enforcement/child protective services

**TABLE 15-1**

## Cutaneous Lesions Often Seen in Abused Children

| Lesion | Likely Cause |
| --- | --- |
| Linear bruising | Striking with a stick or cord |
| Loop-shaped bruising | Striking with a belt or cord |
| Circumferential bruises | Binding injury (e.g., hands tied with rope) |
| Scald injuries in a "stocking/glove" distribution | Submersion in hot water |

| Time Since Injury | Appearance |
| --- | --- |
| 0–2 days | Area swollen and tender |
| 0–5 days | Area red or blue in color |
| 5–7 days | Area green in color |
| 7–10 days | Area yellow in color |
| 10–14 days | Area brown in color |
| 2–4 weeks | Discoloration gone |

(From NMS Pediatrics, 4th ed. Paul H. Dworkin (Ed.). Philadelphia: Lippincott Williams & Wilkins, 2000:70.)

## ❊ Pearls

■ A history of the circumstances of the condition that keeps changing is suspicious for abuse.

■ Children younger than 6 months of age are unable to induce accidents or ingest substances. Be suspicious of bruising in nonambulating infants.

■ Multiplanar injuries are back- and front-sided injuries in combination with left- and right-sided injuries; these injuries are uncommon in true accidents.

- Fractures common in abuse include posterior rib fractures, spinous process fractures, "bucket-handle" fractures, fractures of different ages, multiple bilateral fractures, and complex skull fractures.
- Shaken baby syndrome: retinal hemorrhages, intracranial hemorrhage, rib fractures

## Dyspnea

The presentation of shortness of breath in the pediatric patient can range from such a common condition as a mild cough with tachypnea to the neonate in florid heart failure. A wide differential diagnosis should always be kept. As in pediatric abdominal pain, many diseases are age-specific and can present a diagnostic challenge. The WHO defines tachypnea as ≥60 breaths/min in children 2 months of age or younger, ≥50 breaths/min in children 2–11 months of age, and ≥40 breaths/min in children 12–59 months of age.

### Pertinent Positives/Negatives: OPQRST

- **O**nset: Ask how the dyspnea began, what the child was doing before the symptoms started; determine whether the dyspnea was sudden or insidious in onset and whether there is a history of same condition.
- **P**rovocative/**P**alliative: Determine what makes the dyspnea better or worse (e.g., is it better with albuterol, cold air, moist air, positioning?).
- **Q**uality: grunting, quality of cough (staccato, croupy, whooping, ineffective) (Figure 15-2)

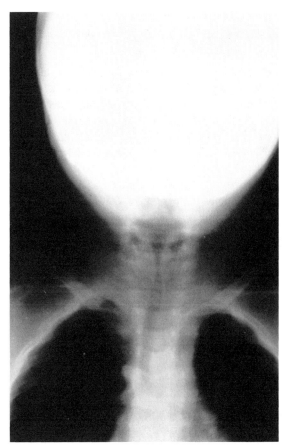

**Figure 15-2** Croup in a 3-year-old. Note the "steeple sign," or the subglottic narrowing, which produces an inverted "V." (*From Mick N, et al. Blueprints Emergency Medicine, 2nd ed. Malden, MA:Blackwell Publishing 2006:217.*)

- **R**egion/**R**adiation: not applicable
- **S**everity: 1 to 10
- **T**iming: constant or intermittent

Miscellaneous: history of asthma, CF, recurrent pneumonias, bronchopulmonary dysplasia, tracheoesophageal fistulas, inborn errors of metabolism, cardiac problems; not acting "right," fevers, decreased appetite, tachypnea, coryza, rashes, abdominal pain, trauma, sick contacts, recent hospital/physician visit, drooling, voice changes, dysphagia, foreign body aspiration, stridor, chest pain, malaise, headaches, conjunctivitis, rhinitis, posttussive emesis, vomiting and/or diarrhea, "blue baby," periods of apnea, exertional dyspnea, feeding intolerance, diaphoresis at midfeeding

 **Physical Examination**

- Fever, tachycardia or bradycardia, hypotension, tachypnea
- Rales, rhonchi, wheezing, consolidation, decreased breath sounds, swollen turbinates, tympanic membrane erythema, pharyngeal exudates/erythema, rashes, visible foreign body, intercostal/subcostal retractions, paradoxical breathing, grunting respirations, abdominal pain, prolonged expiration, periods of apnea, surgical scars, hepatomegaly, generalized edema, cardiac murmurs

 **Laboratory Studies**

- Pulse oximetry, CXR
- Consider CBC, CMP, ECG, blood cultures, RSV/influenza swabs, chest CT

**Management**

- Oxygen (if not contraindicated), albuterol/ipratropium
- Consider steroids/antibiotics, intubation if necessary
- Treat underlying cause

## ✜ Pearls

▦ Apneic episodes can occur with RSV, *Chlamydia*, and pertussis.

▦ "Not all that wheezes is asthma."

## Fever

Fever (defined as rectal temperature of 100.4°F (38.0°C) is one of the most common complaints of infants or children presenting to a physician. Fever can present as part of a clinical presentation ranging from mild benign conditions to severe life-threatening systemic illnesses. Many factors, such as historical facts, physical examination findings, age of the patient, medical history, and immunization status can influence the fever workup. A thorough evaluation should be completed to rule out the serious bacterial infectious causes of fever. One systematic approach to fever in the young patient is to divide the patients into three age groups: younger than 1 month of age, 1–3 months of age, and 3 months of age or older.

### Pertinent Positives/Negatives: OPQRST

▦ **O**nset: Determine when the fever started, how long the fever has been present, and whether it is a subjective fever or one parents measured with a thermometer; check the birth history (for neonate) to look for maternal infections or prematurity.

▦ **P**rovocative/**P**alliative: Ask whether the fever is worse in morning, becomes progressively worse, and whether there has been any recent antibiotic use; ask whether the fever lessens with acetaminophen (Tylenol) or antipyretics (check dose that is being used).

▦ **Q**uality: not applicable

▪ **R**egion/**R**adiation: not applicable
▪ **S**everity: 1 to 10
▪ **T**iming: constant or intermittent

Miscellaneous: associated with poor feeding, vomiting, diarrhea, "uncomfortable," apnea, "not acting right," change in crying/voice, decreased energy, cough, coryza, rash, pain, fatigue, decreased thirst/appetite, recent immunizations, sick contacts (siblings, family members, or recent physician or hospital visit), concomitant medical conditions (immunoglobulin deficiency) , recent travel, "tugging at ear," frequency of urination (hydration status)

### Physical Examination

▪ Fever (measure), tachycardia, tachypnea
▪ Toxic vs. nontoxic appearance, poor social interactions, quality of crying and ease of consolation, presence of tears with crying, fullness of anterior fontanelle, nuchal rigidity, jaundice, rashes (especially hands/feet), skin color, moist mucosa, poor capillary refill, poor eye contact, Kerning sign, Brudzinski sign, grunting, flaring, retractions, "abdominal breathing," abdominal pain, normal gait

### Laboratory Studies (Depend on Age; "Less is More" [i.e., More Workup at Younger Age])

▪ CBC, CMP, UA, CXR, blood cultures, LP with CSF studies
▪ Consider checking for influenza, RSV, streptococcus (rapid strep)

### Management (Fig. 15-3)

▪ Antipyretics, hydration, antibiotics if indicated

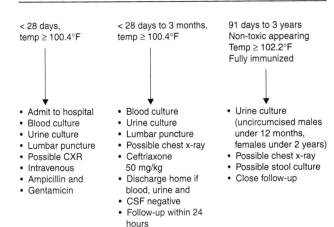

| < 28 days,<br>temp ≥ 100.4°F | < 28 days to 3 months,<br>temp ≥ 100.4°F | 91 days to 3 years<br>Non-toxic appearing<br>Temp ≥ 102.2°F<br>Fully immunized |
|---|---|---|
| • Admit to hospital<br>• Blood culture<br>• Urine culture<br>• Lumbar puncture<br>• Possible CXR<br>• Intravenous<br>• Ampicillin and<br>• Gentamicin | • Blood culture<br>• Urine culture<br>• Lumbar puncture<br>• Possible chest x-ray<br>• Ceftriaxone<br>  50 mg/kg<br>• Discharge home if<br>  blood, urine and<br>• CSF negative<br>• Follow-up within 24<br>  hours | • Urine culture<br>  (uncircumcised males<br>  under 12 months,<br>  females under 2 years)<br>• Possible chest x-ray<br>• Possible stool culture<br>• Close follow-up |

**Figure 15-3** Algorithm for the management of pediatric fever. (*From Mick N, et al. Blueprints Emergency Medicine, 2nd ed. Malden, MA:Blackwell Publishing, 2006:221.*)

## ❇ Pearls

■ Neonates (<28 days of age) who have any documented fever should have a complete workup. (An occult life-threatening event occurs in approximately 1% of children presenting in an acute care setting with fever.)

■ A rectal probe thermometer is most likely to result in an accurate assessment of patient's temperature.

■ Parental reporting of fever on the basis of subjective information is a reliable indicator that fever has been present.

■ Inconsolable crying is frequently seen in infants with meningitis.

■ Children younger than 12 months of age may not show the classic nuchal rigidity, Kerning sign, or Brudzinski sign.

# 16 Psychiatry

## Alcoholism

Alcoholism is both a medical and social problem that has a lifetime prevalence of up to 6%. Up to 20% of all hospital inpatients are alcoholics. Alcoholism can lead to very serious debilitating medical diseases, such as dilated cardiomyopathy, cirrhosis, pancreatitis, GI bleeding, multiple types of cancer, and depression, as well as social harms (DUI, vehicular manslaughter, assault). Be aware that alcohol is often used concomitantly with medications or illicit drugs. Ethanol affects several neurotransmitters in the brain, including opiates, glutamate, serotonin, and GABA, leading to anxiolytic and sedative effects (and explaining the cross-reactivity with benzodiazepines).

### Pertinent Positives/Negatives

- CAGE questionnaire (Have you ever felt the need to **C**ut down on your drinking? Have you ever felt **A**nnoyed by criticism of your drinking? Have you ever felt **G**uilty about drinking? Have you ever had to take an **E**ye opener?). One positive answer makes alcoholism likely.

- Amount of alcohol ingested, illicit drug use, smoking, marital status, previous DUIs/arrests, liver problems, bleeding problems, seizures, hallucinations, depression, suicidal ideation, hematemesis, abdominal pain, pregnancy, family history of alcoholism, last drink of alcohol, previous psychiatric admissions

**Physical Examination**

■ Fever, tachycardia, hypertension, tachypnea

■ AMS, slurred speech, agitation, anxiety, nausea and vomiting, diaphoresis, seizures, delirium, tremors

■ Gynecomastia, testicular atrophy, spider angioma, palmar erythema, ascites, ataxia

 **Laboratory Studies**

■ CBC (with attention to increased MCV/MCH)

■ CMP, liver function tests, BAL, UDS, β-hCG, TSH, PT/INR

 **Management**

■ Treat medical complications

■ Give benzodiazepines for withdrawal/seizures

■ Give multivitamin infusion, thiamine, and folate

■ Provide information about "detox"/alcohol dependence therapy (Alcoholics Anonymous)

❖ **Pearls**

■ If you are giving glucose in a suspected alcoholic patient, give thiamine first to prevent Wernicke encephalopathy.

---

## Bipolar Disorder: Evaluation of the Patient

Bipolar disorder, previously known as manic depression, is divided into two types. Bipolar I disorder is the occurrence of at least one manic episode (with or without psychotic features) that (often) alternates with depressive episodes. Bipolar II disorder is the presence of one hypomanic episode (hypomania is much less severe than full-blown mania). The prevalence of bipolar disorder is approximately 1%, and the condition is more common in adolescents and young adults.

### Symptoms of Bipolar Disorder: DIG FAST

**D**istractibility
**I**nsomnia/**I**ndiscretion
**G**randiosity
**F**light of ideas
**A**gitation/**A**ctivity (increased)
**S**peech (fast/pressured)
**T**houghtlessness

## Pertinent Positives/Negatives

- Excessive spending; indiscriminate sexual activity; misdemeanors, felonies, or traffic tickets; suicidal ideation (passive or active); homicidal ideation; contracts for safety (patient to tell nurse or physician if he or she has suicidal thoughts); specific plan for suicide; past suicide attempts; previous mental illness/diagnoses; access to guns; alcohol use; smoking; illicit drug use; past medical history; thyroid disorders, previous counseling or hospitalization for psychiatric treatment; family history of depression, suicide, or bipolar disorder; living conditions; occupation; education; contraception; hallucinations (visual and auditory); physical or verbal abuse; delusions; current medications (lithium, SSRIs, beta-blockers, thyroid drugs)

## Psychiatric Examination

- Folstein MMSE
- Mental status (alert, lethargic, clouded, somnolent, stuporous), orientation, appearance (neat, tearful, disheveled, tremors), eye contact, attitude (cooperative, uncooperative,

hostile, defensive, agitated, evasive), mood (appropriate, depressed, irritable, euphoric, angry), affect (inappropriate, anxious, flat, blunted, constricted), speech (normal, rapid, slow, monotone, slurred, pressured), judgment, level of motor activity, insight, thought process (flight of ideas, loosening of associations, incoherence, thought blocking), thought content (grandiose, paranoid, religious), sleep disturbances, weight changes (intentional or unintentional)

 **Laboratory Studies**

■ Consider lithium levels, CBC, TSH, RPR, vitamin $B_{12}$, UDS, β-hCG

 **Management**

■ Actively manic: mood stabilizers (lithium, valproate [Depakote])
■ Psychosis: antipsychotics

## 🟥 Pearls

■ Be sure to check for concomitant illicit drug use or a pre-existing medical condition.
■ Be aware of the risks associated with the use of antidepressants in patients with bipolar disorder (mood stabilizers are the first choice).

---

## Depression: Evaluation of the Patient

Major depression is one of the most commonly encountered psychiatric disorders and has a lifetime prevalence of up to 20%. Patients may not present with the lay term "depression" but may have other presenting complaints;

therefore, a high index of suspicion is necessary, and screening questions should be asked. The underlying pathology of depression has not been fully elucidated, but it is theorized that disturbances in serotonin, and possibly norepinephrine and dopamine, levels result in symptoms.

### Symptoms of Depression: SIG E CAPS

**S**leep disturbances
**I**nterests
**G**uilt
**E**nergy
**C**oncentration/memory
**A**ffect/**A**ppetite
**P**sychomotor agitation
**S**uicidal ideation

## Pertinent Positives/Negatives

- Suicidal ideation (passive/active), homicidal ideation, contracts for safety (patient to tell the nurse or physician if he or she has suicidal thoughts), specific plan for suicide, past suicide attempts, previous mental illness/diagnoses, access to guns, alcohol use, smoking, illicit drug use, medical history, thyroid disorders, previous counseling or hospitalization for psychiatric treatment, family history of depression or suicide, living conditions, occupation, education, sexual activity, contraception, hallucinations (visual and auditory), physical or verbal abuse, delusions
- Current medications (SSRIs, beta-blockers, thyroid drugs)

## Psychiatric Examination (Table 16-1)

- Folstein MMSE
- Mental status (alert, lethargic, clouded, somnolent, stuporous), orientation, appearance (neat, tearful, disheveled,

**TABLE 16-1**

## Criteria for Major Depressive Episode

Mood: depressed mood most of the day, nearly every day

Sleep: insomnia or hypersomnia

Interest: marked decrease in interest and pleasure in most activities

Guilt: feelings of worthlessness or inappropriate guilt

Energy: fatigue or low energy nearly every day

Concentration: decreased concentration or increased indecisiveness

Appetite: increased or decreased appetite or weight gain or loss

Psychomotor: psychomotor agitation or retardation

Suicidality: recurrent thoughts of death, suicidal ideation, suicidal plan, suicide attempt

General criteria for a major depressive episode require five or more of the above symptoms to be present for at least 2 weeks; one symptom must be *depressed mood* or *loss of interest or pleasure*. These symptoms must be a change from prior functioning and cannot be due to a medical condition, cannot be substance-induced, and cannot be due to bereavement. The symptoms must also cause *distress or impairment*.

(*Reprinted with permission from American Psychiatric Association. Diagnostic and Statistical Manual of Mental Disorders, 4th ed. Text Revision. 2000.*)

tremors), eye contact, attitude (cooperative, uncooperative, hostile, defensive, agitated, evasive), mood (appropriate, depressed, irritable, euphoric, angry), affect (inappropriate, anxious, flat, blunted, constricted), speech (normal, rapid, slow, monotone, slurred, pressured), judgment, level of motor activity, insight, thought process (flight of ideas, loosening of associations, incoherence, thought blocking), thought content (grandiose, paranoid, religious), sleep disturbances, weight changes (intentional/unintentional)

## Laboratory Studies

■ CBC, TSH, vitamin B$_{12}$, RPR, β-hCG
■ Consider dexamethasone suppression test, serum cortisol, TRH, sleep testing

## Management

■ Pharmacotherapy (SSRIs, TCAs, MAO inhibitors for refractory depression) (Table 16-2)
■ Electroconvulsive therapy (refractory or catatonic depression)
■ Psychotherapy

### TABLE 16-2
#### Antidepressants

**SSRIs**

Citalopram
Fluoxetine
Fluvoxamine
Paroxetine
Sertraline

**Tricyclic Antidepressants**

Amitriptyline
Clomipramine
Desipramine
Doxepin
Imipramine
Nortriptyline

## MAO Inhibitors

Phenelzine
Tranylcypromine

## Other Drugs

Bupropion
Mirtazapine
Nefazodone
Venlafaxine

(*Adapted from Lin TL, Rypkema SW (eds.). Washington Manual of Ambulatory Therapeutics. Philadelphia: Lippincott Williams & Wilkins 2002.*)

## ❌ Pearls

▓ One way to ask about physical or verbal abuse is to ask if the patient feels "safe at home."

▓ "Somatically preoccupied": multiple physically unexplainable complaints (use phrase with caution)

▓ Risk factors for suicide: male sex, ethanol, previous attempt, no significant other, age, depression, rational thoughts, organized plan, recent stressor

## Schizophrenia

Schizophrenia is a syndrome of disturbances of thinking, behavior, and perception. These disturbances must be present for at least 6 months with significant deterioration of social functioning. Schizophrenia manifests in late adolescence or early adulthood. Symptoms can be categorized as positive (delusions, auditory hallucinations, disorganized thought/speech/behavior) or negative (flat affect, social withdrawal, apathy, slow speech) (Table 16-3). The subtypes of schizophrenia are described in Table 16-4. Currently, it is believed

| TABLE 16-3 | |
| --- | --- |
| **Positive and Negative Symptoms of Schizophrenia** | |
| **Negative Symptoms** | **Description** |
| Affective flattening | Decreased expression of emotion, such as lack of expressive gestures |
| Alogia | Literally "lack of words," including poverty of speech and of speech content in response to a question |
| Asociality | Few friends, activities, interests; impaired intimacy, little sexual interest |
| **Positive Symptoms** | |
| Hallucinations | Auditory, visual, tactile, and/or olfactory hallucinations; voices that are commenting |
| Delusions | Often described by content; persecutory, grandiose, paranoid, religious; ideas of reference, thought broadcasting, thought insertion, thought withdrawal |
| Bizarre behavior | Aggressive/agitated, odd clothing or appearance, odd social behavior, repetitive-stereotyped behavior |

(Adapted from Andreasen NC, Black DW. Introductory textbook of psychiatry, 3rd ed. Washington, DC: American Psychiatric Publishing 2001.)

that dopamine overactivity causes the positive symptoms of schizophrenia, whereas serotonin is associated with the negative symptoms.

## Pertinent Positives/Negatives

■ Previous diagnosis of schizophrenia, length of symptoms (family members), family history of schizophrenia, previous head injury, employment history

**TABLE 16-4**

## Subtypes of Schizophrenia

| | |
|---|---|
| Paranoid | Paranoid delusions, frequent auditory hallucination, affect not flat |
| Catatonic | Motoric immobility or excessive, purposeless motor activity, maintenance of a rigid echolalia |
| Disorganized | Disorganized speech, disorganized behavior, flat or inappropriate affect; not catatonic |
| Undifferentiated (probably most common) | Delusions, hallucinations, disorganized speech, catatonic behavior, negative symptoms <br> Criteria not met for paranoid, catatonic, or disorganized |
| Residual | Met criteria for schizophrenia, now resolved, (i.e., no hallucinations, no prominent delusions, but residual negative symptoms or attenuated delusions, hallucinations, or thought disorder) |

*(Adapted from Andreasen NC, Black DW. Introductory textbook of psychiatry, 3rd ed. Washington, DC: American Psychiatric Publishing 2001.)*

■ Hallucinations (auditory or visual), "peculiar" thoughts or habits, mystical or psychic experiences, special powers, anhedonia, delusions (bizarre, such as "God drinks from my nipple," or nonbizarre but unlikely, such as "the police are after me"), medications (especially antipsychotics), compliance with medications, drug use

 **Psychiatric Examination**

■ Folstein MMSE

■ Mental status (alert, lethargic, clouded, somnolent, stuporous), orientation, appearance (neat, tearful, disheveled, tremors), eye contact, attitude (cooperative, uncooperative, hostile, defensive, agitated, evasive), mood (appropriate, depressed, irritable, euphoric, angry), affect (inappropriate, anxious, flat, blunted, constricted), speech (normal, rapid, slow, monotone, slurred, pressured), judgment, level of motor activity, insight, thought process (flight of ideas, loosening of associations, incoherence, thought blocking), thought content (grandiose, paranoid, religious), sleep disturbances, weight changes (intentional/unintentional)

## Laboratory Studies

Consider lithium levels, CBC, TSH, RPR, vitamin $B_{12}$, UDS, β-hCG

## Management

- Atypical antipsychotics treat *both* positive and negative symptoms of schizophrenia.
- Typical antipsychotics treat *only* positive symptoms of schizophrenia.

## Pearls

- Schizophrenia rarely, if ever, manifests initially in the older adult.
- Be aware of neuroleptic malignant syndrome: fever, rigidity, AMS, oculogyric crisis. Discontinue antipsychotic, treat with dantrolene.

# Interpretation of the Chest Radiograph

## General Considerations

The standard chest examination consists of a PA and lateral CXR. The films are read together. The PA film is viewed as if the patient is standing in front of you with his or her right side to your left. The lateral film is viewed as if the patient is facing to the left.

- The PA film is taken in the radiology suite with the patient facing the x-ray cassette. The AP film is used for patients who are unable to be taken to the radiology suite (e.g., those in the ICU and on bed rest, elderly patients, postoperative and trauma cases). On the AP film, the heart is magnified in size. Lateral decubitus films help assess the volume of pleural effusion and demonstrate whether a pleural effusion is mobile or loculated.

- If the exposure is correct:
  - Intervertebral spaces are visible, but vertebrae are not detailed.
  - Bronchovascular structures can usually be seen through the heart.
  - The spine appears to be darker as you move caudally.
  - The sternum should be seen edge on.
  - Two sets of ribs should be visible posteriorly.

- Regarding rotation:
  - The clavicular heads should be equal distance from the vertebral bodies.
  - Rotation can cause the heart and other mediastinal structures to appear enlarged.

## Anatomy

### Normal Erect Posteroanterior Chest x-ray

- Diaphragm at level of the eighth to tenth posterior rib (fifth to sixth anterior rib)
- Vascular markings
  - Pulmonary artery segments and pulmonary veins at mediastinum
  - Gradual decrease in size of vessels more distally
  - Less prominent vasculature in upper lung

### Expiratory Chest x-ray

- Loss of the right heart border silhouette indicates possible pneumonia

### Normal Supine Chest x-ray

- Enlarged cardiac silhouette and ascending aorta
- Vascular markings: Are the upper pulmonary vessels as equally prominent as the lower?

### How to "Read" a Chest x-ray

- Check the name on the x-ray
- Turn off stray lights; optimize room lighting
- Evaluate technique (used by the radiology technician): AP/PA, exposure, rotation, supine or erect

■ Attempt to obtain previous films to use for comparative purposes.

■ Evaluate the entire x-ray systematically; consider using a mnemonic, or working from inside to out or outside to inside. Do not forget to look at all aspects of the x-ray.

### ABCDEFGHI:

**A**orta
**B**ronchus
**C**ord, spinal
**D**iaphragm (look for hyperinflation)
**E**osphagus (look for foreign body)
**F**racture (ribs)
**G**as (look for pneumothorax)
**H**eart (look for cardiomegaly)
**I**atrogenic (subclavian line, pacemaker)

## Findings to Evaluate on Chest x-ray

■ Trachea: midline or deviated, caliber, mass

■ Lungs: abnormal shadowing or lucency

■ Pulmonary vessels: artery or vein enlargement

■ Hila: masses, lymphadenopathy

■ Heart: enlarged (enlarged heart has a width greater than half the width of the entire thorax), mass, mediastinal contour

■ Pleura: effusion, thickening, calcification

■ Bones: lesions or fractures

■ Soft tissues (chest wall, neck): air, with evidence of pneumothorax or tracheobronchial tree injury

■ Diaphragm: free air (free air under the diaphragm is seen in abdominal perforation)

■ ICU films: Identify tubes first and look for pneumothorax.

■ ETT placement: at least 3 cm above the carina

- Central line placement: within the SVC, midway between the azygous vein and right atrium
- NG tube placement: both end and side port in the stomach, projecting over the LUQ (on either CXR or abdominal film)
- Chest tube placement: just anterior to the midclavicular line at the fifth intercostal space, with the distal tip placed superiorly within the pleural space; single radiopaque stripe has a break at the position of the side port that should be in the chest

## Examples of Pathology

### Congestive Heart Failure
- Upper lobe vessels engorged, perihilar haziness
- Interstitial fluid that extends to pleural surfaces
- Kerley B lines, batwing appearance
- Cardiomegaly

### Pneumonia
- Fluffy, patchy, or consolidated
- Does it obscure a heart border or the diaphragm?
- Right upper lobe: anterior/superior location on lateral view
- Right middle lobe
  - Obscures ("silhouettes") border of right side of heart
  - Anterior location on lateral view
- Right lower lobe
  - Obscures right hemidiaphragm but allows visualization of heart border
  - Posterior location on lateral view
- Left upper lobe: lingula
  - Obscures ("silhouettes") border of left side of heart
  - Anterior location on lateral view

■ Left lower lobe
  ■ Obscures left diaphragm
  ■ Posterior location on lateral view

## Pleural Effusion/Hemothorax

■ Blunting of the costophrenic angles
■ If supine: diffuse haziness
■ Lateral decubitus showing layering of fluid
■ Differential diagnosis: CHF, renal failure, tumor, pneumonia, trauma, pancreatitis

## Pneumothorax

■ Air without lung markings
■ Peripheral to the white line of the pleura
■ In an upright film, this is most likely seen in the apices
■ Best demonstrated by an end-expiratory film

## Tension Pneumothorax

■ Air enters the pleural cavity and is trapped during expiration, leading to a buildup of air and increasing intrathoracic pressure, collapsing the lung
■ Mediastinum shifts *away* from the tension pneumothorax (clinically, this can compromise venous filling of the heart)

## Aortic Aneurysm

■ Enlargement of the ascending aorta, arch, or descending aorta
■ Widened mediastinum
■ Left pleural effusion
■ Blurred aortic knob
■ Tracheal or NG tube deviation

- Shift of mainstem bronchus
- Periapical cap

## Emphysema

- Hyperaeration
- Flattened diaphragm
- Long, narrow heart shadow
- Bullae or blebs

## Flail Chest

- Three or more adjacent ribs fractured in two or more places

## Pericardial Effusion

- Enlarged, globular "water bottle"–shaped heart
- Looks like cardiomegaly
- Differential diagnosis: uremia, collagen vascular disease, TB, malignancies, pericarditis

## Pneumomediastinum

- Perforation of GI or respiratory tract
- Air dissecting around the heart or diaphragm into the superior mediastinum

# Appendix B

# Medical Abbreviations

A&O = alert and oriented

AAA = aortic abdominal aneurysm

AACG = acute angle closure glaucoma

AAS = acute abdominal series (x-ray) [chest, supine abdominal, upright x-ray]

ABC = airway, breathing, circulation

ABG = arterial blood gas

ABI = ankle/brachial index

ACE = angiotensin-converting enzyme

ACTH = adrenocorticotropic hormone

ADH = antidiuretic hormone

AF = atrial fibrillation

AFB = acid-fast bacilli

AIDS = acquired immunodeficiency syndrome

ALT = alanine aminotransferase (SGPT)

AMS = altered mental status

ANA = antinuclear antibody

AP = anteroposterior

APD = afferent pupillary defect

ARDS = acute respiratory distress syndrome

ARF = acute renal failure

AS = aortic stenosis

ASA = acetylsalicylic acid

AST = aspartate aminotransferase (SGOT)

AVM = arteriovenous malformation

BAL = blood alcohol level
BC = blood cultures
β-hCG = β-human chorionic gonadotropin
BIPAP = bilevel positive airway pressure
BMP = basic metabolic panel
BNP = B-type natriuretic peptide
BP = blood pressure
BPH = benign prostatic hyperplasia
BPPV = benign paroxysmal positional vertigo
BUN = blood urea nitrogen

CABG = coronary artery bypass graft
CAD = coronary artery disease
CAP = community-acquired pneumonia
CBC = complete blood count
CD4 = cluster of differentiation 4
CF = cystic fibrosis
CHF = congestive heart failure
CMP = complete metabolic profile
CMT = cervical motion tenderness
CNS = central nervous system
COPD = chronic obstructive pulmonary disease
CPAP = continuous positive airway pressure
CPK/MB = cardiac enzymes (CPK = creatine
    phosphokinase)
Cr = creatinine
CRAO = central retinal artery occlusion
CRP = C-reactive protein
CRVO = central retinal vein occlusion
CSF = cerebrospinal fluid
CT = computed tomography
CVA = costovertebral angle, cerebrovascular accident
CVP = central venous pressure
CXR = chest x-ray

D&C = dilation and curettage

$D_5W$ = dextrose 5% in water

DBP = diastolic blood pressure

DDAVP = desmopressin

DHEA-S = dehydroepiandrosterone sulfate

DIC = disseminated intravascular coagulation

DIP = distal interphalangeal (joint)

DKA = diabetic ketoacidosis

DM = diabetes mellitus

DMARD = disease-modifying antirheumatic drug

DPL = diagnostic peritoneal lavage

DRE = digital rectal examination

DUB = dysfunctional uterine bleeding

DUI = driving under the influence (of alcohol)

DVT = deep vein thrombosis

EBV = Epstein-Barr virus

EDH = epidural hematoma

EDTA = ethylenediamine tetraacetic acid

EF = ejection fraction

ECG = electrocardiography, -gram

ELISA = enzyme-linked immunosorbent assay

ENT = ear, nose, throat

ERCP = endoscopic retrograde cholangiopancreatography

ESR = erythrocyte sedimentation rate

ETT = endotracheal tube

$FEV_1$ = forced expiratory volume in 1 second

FFP = fresh-frozen plasma

FHTs = fetal heart tones

FSH = follicle-stimulating hormone

FTA-ABS = fluorescent treponemal antibody
    absorption (test)

FUO = fever of unknown origin

FVC = forced vital capacity

GABA = γ-aminobutyric acid
GBS = Guillain-Barré syndrome
GC = gonorrhea
GCS = Glasgow Coma Scale
GERD = gastroesophageal reflux disease
GGT = gamma-glutamyl transpeptidase
GI = gastrointestinal
GOT = glutamic-oxaloacetic transaminase
GPT = glutamic-pyruvic transaminase

H&P = history and physical examination
hCG = Human Chorionic Gonadrotropin
Hct = hematocrit
HELLP [syndrome] = hemolysis, elevated liver function,
    low platelets
Hgb = hemoglobin
$HgbA_{1C}$ = hemoglobin (glycosylated)
HIDA = hepatobiliary iminodiacetic acid
HIV = human immunodeficiency virus
HLA = human leukocyte antigen
HOCM = hypertrophic obstructive cardiomyopathy
HPF = high-power field
HPI = history of the present illness
HPV = human papilloma virus
HTN = hypertension

ICH = intracranial hemorrhage
ICP = intracranial pressure
ICU = intensive care unit
IDDM = insulin-dependent diabetes mellitus
IHSS = idiopathic hypertrophic subaortic stenosis
INH = isoniazid
INR = international normalized ratio
IOP = intraocular pressure
ITP = idiopathic thrombocytopenic purpura

IUD = intrauterine device
IUP = intrauterine pregnancy
IV = intravenous
IVC = inferior vena cava
IVIG = intravenous immunoglobulin
IVP = intravenous pyelography

JVD = jugular venous distention

KOH = potassium hydroxide

LBO = large bowel obstruction
LDH = lactate dehydrogenase
LE Doppler = low-exposure Doppler
LFT = liver function test
LH = luteinizing hormone
LLQ = left lower quadrant
LMA = laryngeal mask airway
LMP = last menstrual period
LMWH = low-molecular-weight heparin
LOC = loss of consciousness
LP = lumbar puncture
LUQ = left upper quadrant

MAO = monoamine oxidase
MAP = mean arterial pressure
MCH = mean corpuscular hemoglobin
MCP = metacarpophalangeal (joint)
MCV = mean corpuscular volume
MI = myocardial infarction
MMSE = Mini-Mental Status Examination
MONA = Morphine, Oxygen, Nitroglycerin,
    Aspirin
MRI = magnetic resonance imaging
MTX = methotrexate
MVA = motor vehicle accident

NG = nasogastric
NIDDM = non–insulin-dependent diabetes mellitus
NIHSS = National Institutes of Health Stroke Scale
NIPPV = noninvasive positive pressure ventilation
NMS = neuroleptic malignant syndrome
NPO = nothing by mouth
NS = normal saline
NSAID = nonsteroidal anti-inflammatory drug
NSTEMI = non–ST-segment elevation MI
NTG = nitroglycerin

OA = osteoarthritis
OR = operating room

PA = posteroanterior
Pap = Papanicolaou (test)
PCA = patient-controlled analgesia
PCP = *Pneumocystis carinii* pneumonia
PE = pulmonary embolus
PEEP = peak end exploratory pressure
PEFR = peak expiratory flow rate
PFT = pulmonary function test
PID = pelvic inflammatory disease
PIH = pregnancy-induced hypertension
PIP = proximal interphalangeal (joint)
PMI = point of maximum impulse
PND = paroxysmal nocturnal dyspnea
PO = parenteral
POD = postoperative day
PPD = purified protein derivative (Mantoux test)
PPI = proton pump inhibitor
PRBCs = packed red blood cells
PT = prothrombin time
PTCA = percutaneous transluminal coronary
    angioplasty

PTT = partial thromboplastin time
PUD = peptic ulcer disease

RA= rheumatoid arthritis
RBBB = right bundle branch block
RBC = red blood cell
RF = rheumatoid factor
RLQ = right left quadrant
RMSF = Rocky Mountain spotted fever
ROM = range of motion
RPR = Rapid Plasma Reagin
RSV = respiratory syncytial virus
RUQ = right upper quadrant
RVH = right ventricular hypertrophy

SAH = subarachnoid hemorrhage
SARS = severe acute respiratory syndrome
SBO = small bowel obstruction
SBP = systolic blood pressure, spontaneous bacterial
    peritonitis
SCA = sickle cell anemia
SCUBA = self-contained underwater breathing apparatus
SDH = subdural hematoma
SIADH = syndrome of inappropriate antidiuretic hormone
SIRS = systemic inflammatory response syndrome
SLE = systemic lupus erythematosus
$S_3Q_3T_3$ = S wave in lead 1 Q wave in lead 3 inverted T wave
    in lead 3
SSRI = selective serotonin reuptake inhibitor
STD = sexually transmitted disease
STEMI = ST-segment elevation MI
SVC = superior vena cava
SVT = supraventricular tachycardia

TAA = thoracic aortic aneurysm
TB = tuberculosis

TBSA = total body surface area
TCA = tricyclic antidepressant
TEE = transesophageal echocardiography
THC = transhepatic cholangiography
TIA = transient ischemic attack
TPA = tissue plasminogen activator
TRH = thyrotropin-releasing hormone
TSH = thyroid-stimulating hormone
TSS = toxic shock syndrome
TTE = transthoracic echocardiography
TTP = thrombotic thrombocytopenic purpura

UA = urinalysis, unstable angina
UDS = urine drug screen
URI = upper respiratory infection
U/S = ultrasound
UTI = urinary tract infection

VF = ventricular fibrillation
V/Q = ventilation–perfusion
VT = ventricular tachycardia

WBC = white blood cell
WHO = World Health Organization

# Appendix C

# Normal Laboratory Values

**BLOOD, PLASMA, SERUM**

| | |
|---|---|
| Alanine aminotransferase (ALT, GPT at 86°F) | 8–20 U/L |
| Alpha-fetoprotein (AFP) | 0–10 ng/mL |
| Amylase, serum | 25–125 U/L |
| Aspartate aminotransferase (AST, GOT at 86°F) | 8–20 U/L |
| Bilirubin, serum (adult) Total/Direct | 0.1–1.0 mg/dL/ 0.0–0.3 mg/dL |
| Calcium, serum ($Ca^{2+}$) | 8.4–10.2 mg/dL |
| Cholesterol, serum | Recommend: <200 mg/dL |
| Cortisol, serum | 0800 h: 5–23 ng/dL 1600 h: 3–15 ng/dL 2000 h: ≤50% of 0800 h |
| Creatine kinase, serum | Male: 25–90 U/L Female: 10–70 U/L |
| Creatinine, serum | 0.6–1.2 mg/dL |
| Electrolytes, serum Sodium ($Na^+$) Chloride ($Cl^-$) Potassium ($K^+$) Bicarbonate ($HCO_3^-$) Magnesium ($Mg^{2+}$) | 136–145 mEq/L 95–105 mEq/L 3.5–5.0 mEq/L 22–28 mEq/L 1.5–2.0 mEq/L |
| Ferritin, serum | Male: 15–200 ng/mL Female: 12–150 ng/mL |

**BLOOD, PLASMA, SERUM (continued)**

| | |
|---|---|
| Follicle-stimulating hormone, serum/plasma | Male: 4–25 mIU/mL<br>Female:<br>  premenopause:<br>    4–30 mIU/mL<br>  midcycle peak:<br>    10–90 mIU/mL<br>  postmenopause:<br>    40–250 mIU/mL |
| Gases, arterial blood (room air)<br>  pH<br>  $P_{CO_2}$<br>  $P_{O_2}$ | <br>7.35–7.45<br>33–45 mm Hg<br>75–105 mm Hg |
| Glucose, serum | Fasting: 70–110 mg/dL<br>2-h postprandial:<br>  <120 mg/dL |
| Growth hormone-arginine stimulation | Fasting: <5 ng/mL<br>Provocative stimuli:<br>  >7 ng/mL |
| Human chorionic gonadotropin (hCG) | <5 mIU/mL |
| Iron | 50–70 ug/dL |
| Lactate dehydrogenase, serum | 45–90 U/L |
| Luteinizing hormone, serum/plasma | Male: 6–23 mIU/mL<br>Female:<br>  follicular phase<br>    5–30 mIU/L<br>  midcycle<br>    75–150 mIU/mL<br>  postmenopause<br>    30–200 mIU/mL |
| Osmolality, serum | 275–295 mOsmo/kg |
| Parathyroid hormone, serum, N-terminal | 230–630 pg/mL |

**BLOOD, PLASMA, SERUM (continued)**

| | |
|---|---|
| Phosphate (alkaline), serum (p-NPP at 30°C) | 20–70 u/L |
| Phosphorus (inorganic), serum | 3.0–4.5 mg/dL |
| Prolactin, serum (hPRL) | <20 ng/mL |
| Prostate-specific antigen | 0–4 ng/mL |
| Proteins, serum | |
| Total, recumbent | 6.0–7.8 g/dL |
| Albumin | 3.5–5.5 g/dL |
| Globulin | 2.3–3.5 g/dL |
| Testosterone, serum | 300–1,000 ng/dL |
| Thyroid-stimulating hormone, serum or plasma | 0.5–5.0 nU/mL |
| Thyroidal iodine ($^{123}$I) uptake | 8%–30% of administered dose/24h |
| Thyroxine ($T_4$), serum | 5–12 ng/dL |
| Triglycerides, serum | 35–60 mg/dL |
| Triiodothyronine ($T_3$), serum (RIA) | 115–190 ng/dL |
| Triiodothyronine ($T_9$), resin uptake | 25%–35% |
| Urea nitrogen, serum (BUN) | 7–18 mg/dL |
| Uric acid, serum | 3.0–8.2 mg/dL |

**HEMATOLOGIC**

| | |
|---|---|
| Bleeding time (template) | 2–7 minutes |
| Erythrocyte count | Male: 4.3–5.9 million/mm$^3$ Female: 3.5–5.5 million/mm$^3$ |

**HEMATOLOGIC (continued)**

| | |
|---|---|
| Erythrocyte sedimentation rate (Westergren) | Male: 0–15 mm/h<br>Female: 0–20 mm/h |
| Hematocrit | Male: 41%–53%<br>Female: 36%–46% |
| Hemoglobin A1C | ≤6% |
| Hemoglobin, blood | Male: 13.5–17.5 g/dL<br>Female: 12.0–16.0 g/dL |
| Leukocyte count and differential | |
|     Leukocyte count | 4,500–11,000/mm$^3$ |
|     Segmented neutrophils | 54%–62% |
|     Bands | 3%–5% |
|     Eosinophils | 1%–3% |
|     Basophils | 0%–0.75% |
|     Lymphocytes | 25%–33% |
|     Monocytes | 3%–7% |
| Mean corpuscular hemoglobin | 25.4–34.6 pg/cell |
| Mean corpuscular hemoglobin concentration | 31%–36% Hb/cell |
| Mean corpuscular volume | 80–100 fl |
| Partial thromboplastin time (activated) | 25–40 seconds |
| Platelet count | 150,000–400,000/mm$^3$ |
| Prothrombin time | 11–15 seconds |
| Reticulocyte count | 0.5%–1.5% of red cells |
| Thrombin time | <2 seconds deviation from control |
| Volume | |
|   Plasma | Male: 25–43 mL/kg<br>Female: 28–45 mL/kg |
|   Red cell | Male: 20–36 mL/kg<br>Female: 19–31 mL/kg |

**URINE**

| | |
|---|---|
| Calcium | 100–300 mg/24 h |
| Chloride | Varies with intake |
| Creatine clearance | Male: 97–137 mL/min |
| | Female: 88–128 mL/min |
| Osmolality | 50–1,400 mOsmol/kg |
| Oxalate | 8–40 ng/mL |
| Potassium | Varies with diet |
| Proteins, total | <150 mg/24 h |
| Sodium | 40–220 mEq/24 h |
| Uric acid | 210–750 mg/24 h |

**URINALYSIS**

| | |
|---|---|
| Color | Clear |
| Odor | None |
| Glucose | None |
| Ketones | None |
| Protein | <150 mg/24 h |
| pH | 4.5–8.0 |
| Specific gravity | 1.001–1.035 |
| Red cells | 0–3 HPF |
| White cells | 0–3 HPF |
| Bacteria | Negative |
| Crystals | Negative |
| Epithelial cells | Not significant |

**SEMINAL FLUID ANALYSIS**

| | |
|---|---|
| Appearance | Opaque, gray-white, highly viscid |
| Volume | 2–5 mL |
| Liquefaction | Complete within 30 minutes |
| pH | 7.2–8.0 |

**SEMINAL FLUID ANALYSIS** (continued)

| | |
|---|---|
| Leukocytes | Occasional or absent |
| Count | 20–250 million/mL |
| Motility | 50%–80% with progressive active motility |
| Morphology | 50%–90% with normal forms |

# Dermatomes

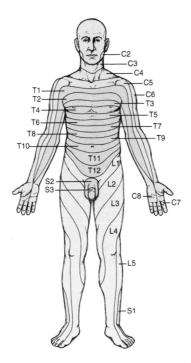

(*Continued*)

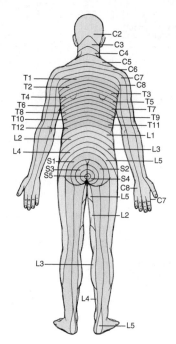

**D-1** Distribution of Dermatomes on the Skin. (*From Stedman's Medical Dictionary, 27th ed. Baltimore: Lippincott Williams & Wilkins., 2000.*)

# Index

Page numbers followed by *f* or *t* refer to figures or tables, respectively.